NICU Nursing Stories

NICU NURSING STORIES

A Day in the Life of a NICU Nurse

VALERIE WRIGHT, DNP, RN, CNE, CHSE, RYT

Illinois State University

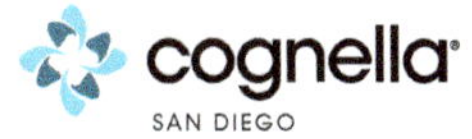

Bassim Hamadeh, CEO and Publisher
Amanda Martin, Publisher
Amy Smith, Senior Project Editor
Rachel Kahn, Production Editor
Jess Estrella, Senior Graphic Designer
Kylie Bartolome, Licensing Associate
Natalie Piccotti, Director of Marketing
Kassie Graves, Senior Vice President, Editorial

Printed in the United States of America.

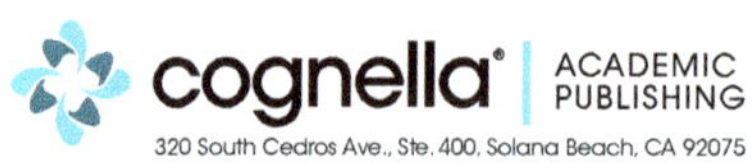

This book is dedicated to all the babies and their families I was privileged to care for while working as a nurse in the NICU. I will forever be in awe of their strength, tenacity, resilience, and love. And to my precious twins, Joey, and Callie. I am thankful God chose me to be your mommy. You will never be forgotten.

Contents

Acknowledgments

Proverbs 3:6 says, "In all your ways acknowledge Him, and He will make your paths straight." Without the grace and mercy of God, I wouldn't be on a "path" at all, much less writing this book. I have been through some pretty dark paths in my life, and despite it all, God continued to speak light and love into my heart and soul. The fact that I can remember these stories with such clarity is nothing short of a miracle—a true gift from God. I look forward to the day when I can give Him the biggest high-five ever! God—you are the snazziest of all!

I am forever indebted to my husband, Kevin, for his love and support and for believing in me throughout this entire endeavor, even on the days I did not believe in myself. From the bottom of my heart, thank you.

To my youngest stepson, Philip, your support, even when you didn't know you were giving it, has been invaluable. From the moment I married your father, you embraced the memory of Joey and Callie. I cannot tell you how much that meant to me. Now that you're all grown up, you have gone above and beyond to create a priceless treasure to store Joey and Callie's ashes. Whenever I see the beautifully welded tree in the shape of a heart, I am reminded of God's promises that He will never leave or forsake us. Philip, thank you for always being there.

A heartfelt thanks to my parents and step-parents, sisters, and extended family. Not only did you walk alongside me through some of the darkest moments of my life, but you have also been there to cheer me on in the good times. God blessed me with an amazing family, and I cannot thank you enough for all you have done and continue to do for me.

To my college roommate and best friend, Kim. You have stuck by me through it all. You dropped everything to be with me in the ICU and would do the same today if needed.

While our physical locations separate us, we continue to share an unbreakable bond. And to my best friend, Heidi, although we've only known each other for a few years, it feels like we've been friends for a lifetime. Your constant support, prayers, and encouragement throughout this entire process have been invaluable. Kim and Heidi, you are the best friends ever, and I am so thankful God placed you both on my path.

To all my friends at Bayle's Lake for always checking in and being so very supportive. It is almost as if God placed you all near me as encouraging cheerleaders to be with me throughout this entire book-writing process. Thanks for being the best neighbors I could ever ask for!

To my dog and very best furry friend, Jäger. Although you'll never be able to read this, it didn't feel right to leave you out. Even as I write out this acknowledgment section, you are by my side. Somehow you always knew when I needed you and your sweet puppy kisses. I love you, bubby.

To the staff and my friends at Sol Hot Yoga, Matt, Sky, and Jenni. I specifically stayed at a location near your studio when writing the book because I knew I would need the very best yoga a studio could ever offer. You provided space for me to work through the emotions that bubbled up as I wrote out story, after story, after story. Namaste, my friends.

To all the peer reviewers and editors who spent their time and energy reviewing this book. Your contributions helped make this book better than I could have imagined.

To all the staff at Cognella who helped make my dream a reality. Specifically, Amanda, Amy, Rachel, and Jess. Amanda, I still remember our first conversation when you asked for me to write a book on Nursing Leadership, to which I said, "No thank you; however, I do have another idea." You were open to the idea of this book from the beginning. Thank you for believing in me and my dream of writing this book. Amy and Rachel, I cannot thank you enough for your countless hours of support during this writing process. You helped guide me each step of the way, which I truly appreciate. To Jess, I had no idea what would happen with the cover design, but somehow, you took what was in my mind and made it far better than I could ever have imagined. Ladies—you all ROCK!

Many thanks to my coworkers in the NICU who endured countless hours of Enya and were my fierce supporters after Joey and Callie died. I was fortunate to work alongside such supportive and compassionate colleagues whose commitment to providing quality, evidence-based care to our tiniest patients is outstanding.

My sincerest thanks to all the contributing authors in this book. Thank you for your time and dedication to writing a story/stories about your own time in the NICU. Remembering the story is one thing, but writing it is an entirely different endeavor. Your contributions helped to make this book what it is today, and for that, I am very grateful.

A special thanks to Evelyn Nuss (1932–2009) whose legacy lives on in her two children, Tim and Kim Nuss. Thank you for keeping letters from first graders and taking the time and energy to mail them out when they graduated years later. I would also like to acknowledge the teachers I have had throughout my years of school. From elementary all the way to my doctor of nursing practice, each of you has played a special role in helping me to be the person I am today. There are too many names to mention, but you know who you are. Thank you.

Last but not least, I would like to thank all the babies and their families I was privileged to care for while working as a nurse in the NICU. A special thanks to those who gave me permission to tell your specific story. I underestimated the weight I would feel as I attempted to write out the story of your precious children. I pray I was able to write them in a way that you each find meaningful. What an honor it has been to not only care for your babies but also write about my experiences. God placed each of you on my path, and I am forever grateful for that gift.

Contributors

Laura Bowgren, BSN, RN

Kelli Daugherty, MSN, APRN, CNM

Jennifer Rigdon, BSN, RN, CRHCP

Diedra Stewart, MSN, CNL, CLC

Linda Jo Swartz, RNC

Kathey Voelker, RNC, NNP

Christine Wetzel, DNP, RNC-NICU, IBCLC

Mary Jayne Zonfrilli, NNP-BC

Reviewers

Pamela Smith, MSN, FNP-BC, RNC-NIC
Assistant Professor of Nursing
Carson-Newman University

Stacey Sears, DNP, CPNP-AC
Wayne State University College of Nursing

Barb McClaskey, PhD, RNC-NICU
Pittsburg State University

Brenda K. Batts, MPH-RRT, NPS-RRT
Assistant Professor and Program Director,
Cardiorespiratory Science
Tennessee State University

Chris Wetzel, DNP, RNC-NIC, IBCLC
Adjunct Faculty at University of Illinois Chicago,
College of Nursing, Urbana Campus
Evidence-Based Practice Specialist,
Carle Hospital NICU, Urbana, Illinois

Introduction

From the moment I knew I could "be" something when I grew up, I knew I wanted to be a neonatal intensive care unit (NICU) nurse, so much so that when my class's first-grade teacher asked us to write what we wanted to be when we grew up, I wrote, "I want to be a nurse and work with babies, and I hate math." I know this because my first-grade teacher, Mrs. Evelyn Nuss, sent me the letter I wrote when I graduated high school. She did this for all the students she had, year after year. It is something I will always treasure.

After graduating high school, I attended nursing school at the Mennonite College of Nursing. I was in the last class to graduate from the private college before it became a part of Illinois State University. My career has taken me to many places, but ultimately, it has ended up where it all began, except now I am a nurse educator at Mennonite College of Nursing and not a nursing student. However, I would argue that I will always be a student, as I can never stop learning about this amazing nursing profession.

Nursing school was hard—at times, almost impossible. However, with the support of my family and friends, faculty, much determination, and the grace of God, I made it through, graduating summa cum laude. You see, it was hard because I only ever wanted to take care of babies, and nursing school was filled with mostly adults. If my memory serves me correctly, I believe I had one lecture on NICU care, and that was it, out of hours and hours of nursing school. I was also a hot mess at clinical. I cried before every clinical, except the few I had on the obstetric unit. I am pretty sure the faculty played "rock, paper, scissors" to decide who had to have me in their clinical.

While in nursing school, I had the opportunity to take a special elective that I was able to design. So, of course, I designed it around the NICU. I even found a faculty member who worked in a nearby NICU willing to allow me to shadow her for a week. My first day as a student in the NICU finally came, and I couldn't have been more excited! Little did I know that it would be much more challenging than I expected.

I vividly remember watching a NICU nurse putting an IV in a baby's scalp. Due to my lack of knowledge, I thought she was putting it into their brain. I had never seen anything like it. I felt a rush of warmth come over my body, and the next thing I knew, I was in the nurse's lounge with a giant bump on my head. I had passed out cold at the baby's bedside. My instructor was so kind as she dealt with me freaking out about how "now I can't be a NICU nurse because I can't 'hack' it." She reassured me that seeing a scalp IV was an intense thing to witness and informed me that it wasn't going into the baby's brain. I thought my dream was over, but thankfully, it wasn't.

When it came time to graduate and apply for jobs, I discovered that the hospital I lived near did not hire new graduates into the NICU. I was devastated. I had made it through what, at the time, were the hardest four years of my life, and now I wasn't going to get to do what I had dreamed about since the first grade. Enter Plan B. The obstetrical (OB) unit was hiring, so I applied and was offered a night shift position as a postpartum and newborn nursery RN, which I eagerly took. For those in nursing school reading this, your first job might not be your dream job. It might not even be close, but don't let that frustrate you, because I promise it is all part of a bigger plan.

Working in postpartum and newborn nursery taught me a lot about normal newborn care. This gave me an advantage as a NICU nurse, as I could spot abnormalities much quicker. I was also able to refine my skills as a nurse in a fairly stable environment. I would never have voluntarily taken that job, but in hindsight, it was probably the best thing to have happened to me. Even though the job was good for me, I took every chance I could to go to the NICU. After a while, they needed help, and I volunteered. I did everything extra I could in the NICU, praying it would help gain me the coveted position as a NICU RN. After nine months of working in postpartum and newborn nursery, I was offered a full-time night shift position as a NICU RN, and I never looked back.

The night shift was not kind to my body, but I loved the NICU, and the night shift was the only option at the beginning. I worked just shy of 5 years of nights before a day position became available, which I gladly took. I learned so much on the night shift. In fact, many of the stories in this book come from my time on nights. I believe Charles Dickens summed up my time on the night shift well when he said:

> It was the best of times, it was the worst of times, it was the age of wisdom, it was the age of foolishness, it was the epoch of belief, it was the epoch of incredulity, it was the season of light, it was the season of darkness, it was the spring of hope, it was the winter of despair.[1]

I worked as a staff and transport nurse as well as a charge nurse on the night shift. This continued when I transitioned to the day shift. After several years, I became a shift supervisor and, ultimately, moved into the interim nurse manager role. I had worked my way "up the ladder," but ultimately, it took me farther from what I loved, which was caring for the babies and teaching new nurses how to do the same. Once Kevin and I were married, the long hours I was working conflicted with our family time. He had three boys, and time was going by so quickly. I was missing out on many of the boys' events, which weighed heavily on my heart.

The last straw was when I promised my middle stepson that I would be at his band concert. Don't get me wrong, I was not excited about a junior high band concert, but I was excited to see *him* perform. However, I missed it due to an emergency in the NICU. As a nurse, you cannot just walk away during a code situation (when the baby isn't breathing, and their heart has stopped beating). I arrived at the concert to hear the last note played. I will never forget him asking me if I saw the entire thing and then the despair on his face when I told him the truth about how I had just arrived. I did not want this to happen again. God had given me a gift with these three boys, and I wasn't going to squander it away working 60- to 70-hour weeks.

---

1 Charles Dickens, *A Tale of Two Cities* (London: James Nisbet, 1902), 3.

After much prayer and thoughtful discussion with my husband, I returned to school to get my master of science in nursing (MSN) in nursing education. After graduating, I worked as the perinatal educator in our Nursing Education department. I stayed in that position for a few years and then received a job offer to be the director of nursing at a local community college. I interviewed but planned to say no. However, the office was painted pink and was warm (I am always cold). I took these things as a sign from God that I was supposed to be there.

I stayed in that position for two years and then advanced my career to being the associate dean of nursing at another community college. I was in that position for 3 years before I finally came back "home" to my alma mater, Mennonite College of Nursing. I also went back to school, for the *last* time, to get my doctor of nursing practice (DNP) degree. Now, I have the opportunity to teach hundreds of nursing students each year. In class, I tell several of the stories I have written, which ultimately gave me the idea to write this book. This was my way of having these stories live on forever for any student to read, not just the ones I am privileged to teach.

In writing this book, I collaborated with several contributing authors. These authors were nurses I had the honor of working with in the NICU, and to this day, I still consider them my friends. I can't thank them enough for their time and dedication in sharing their precious stories, which you can find in Part II of this book. The other exciting thing about writing this book is that I had the opportunity to help design the cover. The nurse on the cover is representative of all the nurses out there who have cared for patients. Regardless of where nurses work, the interactions with their patients and families can sometimes be very heavy. The nurse on the cover is all of us. Additionally, the footprints on the mask are those of my twins, Joey and Callie, which you will get to read in the story titled "It Is Well With My Soul." Joey's footprints are on the left and Callie's on the right. They were placed in a specific area on the nurse's mask to represent tears. Sometimes, those tears are happy tears, and sometimes, they are tears from extreme heartache. As nurses, we give a little piece of ourselves to each patient we have the privilege of caring for, and I hope that spirit is represented within the cover of this book.

I also want to acknowledge that the stories I wrote are written from my own personal memory of the experience. Memories are an interesting thing. I can be at the same event as someone else, yet we remember it completely differently. With that said, if you were involved in these stories and remember them differently, I completely understand. It was my intention to write them with the accuracy with which I remembered them, and I hope I did just that. Additionally, some names have been changed, as I am no longer in touch with their family. However, many of the names you will read are the actual names of the babies I cared for—a special thanks to their parents for allowing me to write about their precious babies.

This book was written to cover a wide audience. I hope healthcare professionals, especially nurses and nursing students, can connect to the stories and how they might relate to their own professional practice. I also hope individuals from the general public can get a glimpse of what it was like in the NICU. Furthermore, this book was not written assuming that the reader would start at the beginning and read through to the end. This book was intentionally designed to pick up and read, perhaps just one story at a time. So, feel free to break all the "rules" of standard book reading. You might conceivably start with a story from "Unforgettable NICU Stories," then move to a story from a contributing author, and finish with a story from "The Lighter Side of the NICU." There are no rules.

This is your book to read how you would like. However, I recommend reviewing the reflection questions at the end of each story and perhaps even the reflective journaling at the end of the book. The stories written in this book could bring up an array of emotions for you as you read them. These reflection questions will allow space for you to process the events and corresponding emotions that may have sprung up throughout the book. Your feelings are just as real as the feelings of the authors of this book. If you find yourself struggling, whether it be mentally or emotionally, as you read the book, please reach out for help.

I have been teaching since 2008 and have loved *almost* every minute. While I miss the babies in the NICU, I do not miss the hours, the weekends, the holidays, the mandatory call, or the emotional stress from watching a precious baby die in their parent's arms. I thank God for every second I spent with the babies and their families in the NICU. I carry a part of them with me in all that I do. Their story is a permanent part of my story, which I am forever grateful for. As you read the following stories, may you gain a small insight into what a day in the life of a NICU nurse is like.

Correspondence with the author can be done through nicunursingstories@gmail.com.

PART I

It Is Well With My Soul

It Is Well With My Soul

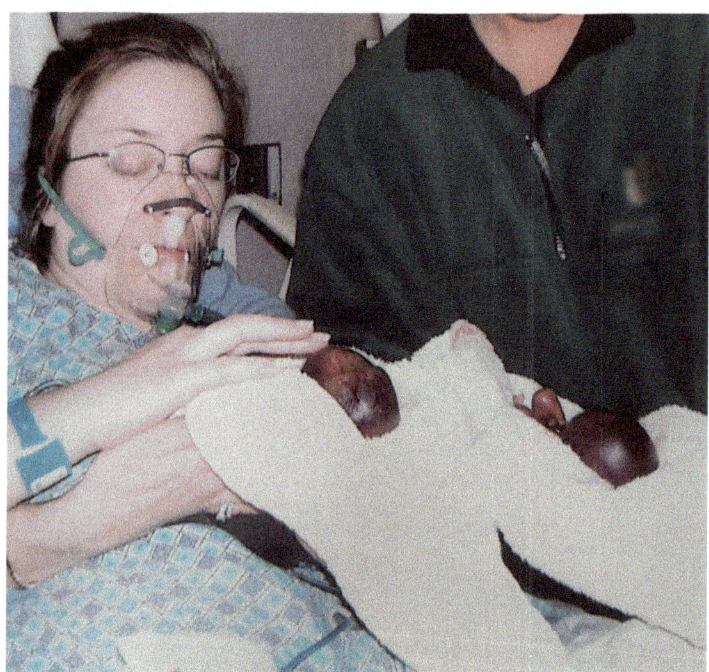

IMG 1.1

This story is a bit harder to write, mainly because it is my personal story. It all started in 2000 when my husband Richard and I had been trying to have a baby on our own for a year and were transitioning to seeing an infertility specialist. I had endometriosis, which caused issues with us getting pregnant. Little did we know we would embark on 6 years of infertility before getting pregnant for the first and only time.

After two surgeries and countless failed attempts to get pregnant, we decided to do in vitro fertilization (IVF). IVF is a process where the sperm fertilizes the egg outside of the body, and then once the embryos form, they are placed back into the uterus. We had terrible luck in the past, so the fact that the process went really well was rather shocking. We had several good embryos and decided to implant two and freeze the rest.

Once I got home from the hospital, I laid down to nap. Our sweet and sassy Chihuahua, Skeeter Bug, always slept with us at the foot of the bed—under the covers, of course. However, that day was different. When she snuggled down to the foot of the bed, she did her usual three circles and then got up and moved toward my belly, where she did three more circles and then laid down to have her nap. At the time, I thought it was really odd that she would do that, as she had never done that before. I think back then and wonder if she knew I was pregnant. She slept by my belly each night until my water broke and I went into the hospital. I loved that she did that.

The pregnancy went remarkably well. I was sick at the beginning with morning sickness, but luckily it didn't last much into the second trimester. My husband was getting ready to go out of town, which was odd for him, as he usually didn't travel. He had a goal of having the nursery done before he left, and done it was. The walls were painted, cribs and dressers were put together, and we were starting to decorate the walls. The decorations were going to be inspired by Noah's Ark. The theme of "two by two" seemed fitting for a room for twins. The only thing missing was the rocking chair. I had my eye on a beautiful pink (I *love* pink) plush rocking chair, which my dad had agreed to purchase for the twins and me. The chair had to be specially ordered, so it was on its way.

The day I took my husband to the airport was my last 12-hour shift at the hospital. Because I am on the smaller side (5 ft 0 inches, 100 lbs), there wasn't much room for the babies, so my belly grew quickly. I actually measured full-term at 20 weeks, so people who didn't know me thought I was ready to deliver a full-term baby. I was going to move to 4- and 8-hour shifts because it was getting more challenging for me to get around and my doctor wanted to be on the safe side. When I dropped him off at the airport, I cried. I had this impending sense of doom that made no sense. I begged him not to go, which was weird because I would usually be excited to have just a few days to myself. He reassured me everything was going to be okay and boarded his plane.

I worked my last 12-hour shift and then went home. My neighbor (and friend) had made me supper (because cooking after a 12-hour shift sucks), and then I went home to bed. I woke up around 5 a.m. to my water breaking in my bed. I immediately sat up and screamed. I ran to the bathroom as amniotic fluid was gushing out everywhere. Then I called the labor and delivery (L&D) department of the hospital and talked to one of the nurses (who was also one of my friends) and told her what happened. She reassured me that I had probably just "peed the bed" and that I was fine. I explained that it was not urine. I could also feel my belly had dropped, likely because there was less fluid inside. She said to come in and she would check me but that she'd probably end up just sending me back home. To this day, I wish she had been right.

I was distraught, and there was no way I could drive. I called my friend, who was also the neighbor across the street. She rushed across the street and drove me to the hospital. From the moment I arrived, I was not okay. Unfortunately, I was correct. My son's amniotic sac had broken, and my daughter's sac was still intact. I was actively contracting. I knew it wasn't good, as I was 21 and 6/7 weeks pregnant the day I was admitted. Babies are considered "viable" at 24 weeks. At that time, babies could survive between 23 and 24 weeks, but their outcomes, if they survived, were not good. However, babies under 23 weeks simply couldn't survive. Technology wasn't advanced enough to handle their undeveloped lung sacks and other micro preemie needs. However, today, with the help of technology, advanced science, and amazing NICU staff, babies at 22 weeks have a chance for survival, which you will read about in the story "The Miracle of Birth" by Dr. Christine Wetzel.

They called my husband, and he rushed to get the first flight back home. Meanwhile, they had trouble stopping the contractions, so they had to increase the medicine (magnesium sulfate). Despite being on the maximum dose, I was still contracting. As the day progressed into night, I became sicker. I ended up having a fever of 106° and was shaking uncontrollably. It was horrible. At that time, they had drawn labs that were positive for an infection, specifically *E. coli* sepsis. They decided to take me off the medicine to stop contractions and put me on medication to start contractions (pitocin). What a weird thing for my body to go through. It must have been thinking, "Y'all need to get your story straight—first, we aren't supposed to contract, and now you want us to? Make up your mind."

When my temperature was so high, the nurse came in with a bucket of ice water and asked my husband to take washcloths and move them around my body. He was supposed to put them around my legs, arms, neck, and face. To hear him tell the story (because I was out of it at this point), he says that he went back and told the nurse he needed another bucket. "If I use the same bucket 'down there' on her face, even though she seems out of it, she will know. I guarantee it." I'm unsure if I would have known, but I am glad he advocated for the second bucket. I have always been a germ "freak."

My entire family had also come to the hospital to provide support, as they understood the gravity of the situation. In hindsight, I believe they understood the potential outcome for Joey and Callie but had no idea that I might also lose my life. My family stayed around the clock, sometimes in my room and other times in the waiting lounge. They also assisted with the ice bath to get my temperature to lower into a normal range. One of my sisters commented on how her hands were so cold she couldn't feel them, but she continued, as she felt like that was the only thing she could do to help. I cannot imagine how helpless they must have felt watching me go through what I did.

At some point in the middle of all of this, they took me to get an ultrasound. They were trying to see if they could deliver Joey and keep Callie inside until she was old enough to survive. The sonogram was a vague memory, almost like a dream and not my actual reality. My family had gone with me to the sonogram. To hear them tell the story, I was "completely out of it," which absolutely broke their hearts. They knew they were watching Joey's heartbeat for the last time and wished that I would also be able to experience that moment.

Unfortunately, one of the earliest signs of sepsis is a change in mental status known officially as sepsis-associated delirium. I apparently was asking for my tea as they did their best to hold back tears. I am not sure I could have been as strong as they were.

Back in labor and delivery, the contractions became more intense, and I got sicker. My lungs began filling with fluid, and each breath I took became harder and harder. I remember the obstetrician telling me I would be transferred to the ICU once I delivered the twins. I specifically asked if I could go to the NICU because the adult ICU was "gross." I told her, "I'm small. I can fit in those cribs. Plus, I know the nurses." Clearly, this wasn't going to happen, but I also didn't think it would happen that I would have to go to the adult ICU. I figured she was being cautious. Little did I know I would actually be admitted to the adult ICU, where I would be fighting for my life.

I had been given a Willow Tree figurine when going through infertility. The figurine held up the word "hope" between her hands. I had kept it at my bedside at home, as it was a great reminder to have hope in a hopeless circumstance. My friend had brought that figurine to the hospital and placed it on top of my IV pump so I could see it and be reminded to have hope. However, one of the L&D nurses had entered my room and accidentally bumped it. It fell to the floor and shattered. Not even the figurine had hope anymore.

As my lungs began filling with fluid, my oxygen saturation began dropping. They kept putting me on a non-rebreather mask with oxygen (a face mask connected to a reservoir bag that's filled with a high concentration of oxygen), which I would promptly remove. Because you see, in delivery, when the mom is put on oxygen, it is for the baby, not the mom. I knew my babies would not survive, so I didn't need that annoying mask. In hindsight (after reviewing my chart), my oxygen saturation was dropping into the 50s, thus the actual need for oxygen for *my* lungs.

When you know the rules, you know how to break them—and break them, I did. I didn't tell the nurses my lungs were filling up with fluid. I knew if I told them, they would do an emergency C-section and I wouldn't get to hold my twins. So, I kept that little secret to myself. The time came for me to deliver them; it took everything I had.

Our son, Joey Thomas, was born on March 2, 2006, at 3:00 p.m. He weighed 444 grams (15.7 ounces), just shy of one pound. When I was admitted to the hospital, he had a heartbeat, but by the time I delivered, he did not. He was born perfect and still.

A few minutes later, at 3:23 p.m., our daughter, Callie Marie, was born. She weighed 376 grams (13.3 ounces). She let out the tiniest cry when she was born, and we had the opportunity to hold her for the few precious moments she was alive on this Earth. She took her last breath in our arms. We baptized the babies, surrounded by our family and friends. It was horrific and perfect all at the same time.

It was as if my body knew I had accomplished what I wanted to do—to hold Joey and Callie in my arms—because immediately after they were baptized, my body began shutting down. The placentas wouldn't release, so I was also bleeding to death on top of going into organ failure. They took me back to the operating room (OR) for an emergency dilation and curettage (D&C) to surgically remove the placentas from the uterus. I barely breathed when sitting upright, so lying on the flat operating room table made matters significantly worse. I still remember people running all around in a panic. It was mass chaos in that operating room. Emergencies involving maternal sepsis and the complications associated with it are statistically rare occurrences, and rarely, if ever, do they happen to one of their own. I had been in that OR multiple times as the nurse, just never as the patient.

As I was lying on the table, I heard the anesthesiologist click the laryngoscope blade (a blade used to assist with intubation, which is putting a tube into the patient's throat and down into their lungs). It makes a very specific sound that I was quite familiar with. I thought to myself, "Surely, he will sedate me before he intubates me." Unfortunately, I was wrong. He tried to intubate me without sedation, so I quickly hit the laryngoscope out of his hand, which clearly irritated him. He told the nurse (one of my friends) to "tie me down." (The OR table has straps for the arms, and the nurse hadn't strapped my arms down because I was already struggling to breathe.)

He then attempted to intubate me again; however, I still was not sedated, and bonus: The nurse only tied one arm down. So, I waited for him to get really close, and then with all my might, I punched him in the face. If he was irritated before, he was in a full-on rage now. He yelled at the nurse to strap me down and hold me still so he could intubate me. As if breathing wasn't hard enough, the nurse laid across me and held my head still. I can still feel her tears falling onto my face as she said, "I'm so sorry, Valerie. I'm so sorry."

But guess what? All the holding in the world doesn't prevent me from biting down so that he can't get in my mouth. Knowing this would not happen, I heard him open the "magical" medication box filled with many "good" drugs to knock me out. Thank goodness! Finally! Except, he only used the medication to paralyze me, not the one to sedate me. So, I could feel, see, and hear everything, but I couldn't move, as I was completely paralyzed. What seemed like an eternity of hell likely lasted less than a minute because I didn't remember anything else once I was intubated and placed on the ventilator.

I had always thought that being intubated awake would be torturous. Never did I imagine one of my worst nightmares coming true. I later asked my best friend Kim, a certified registered nurse anesthetist (CRNA), why they would have done that. She explained that because my blood pressure was so low, as well as my oxygenation, they likely didn't use sedation out of fear of it dropping more, and they would have thought I wouldn't remember because my oxygen was so low. But guess what? I remember.

After that, they did the emergency D&C, and I became more unstable. They planned to stabilize me in the OR before transporting me to the ICU, but I only got worse. Meanwhile, it had been a while since they had updated my family. My mom, who is just as sassy as me, found a way to get into the OR, where they explained what was happening. My husband was waiting with one of our neonatologists in a different area of the hospital. The neonatologist took my husband back to the OR to see me. Because of the chaos, nobody said anything to my husband. He looked at me, my eyes swollen shut, my skin grey and cold, and wondered if I had already died. He saw the monitors, heard all the beeping, and took that as a positive sign.

He followed the staff alongside me to the ICU. He said he knew it was a good thing when they pressed the "up" button rather than the "down" button on the elevator (he knew the morgue was in the basement). Once I got to the ICU, I became even more critical. My family and friends said the doctors came to the waiting room to get them. They said the doctors had relayed how critical I was and that it was time for them to say their final goodbyes. I cannot imagine what that must have been like for them.

Spoiler alert: I am the one writing this story, and apparently, God wasn't done with my life story! I was on a ventilator in the ICU on maximum settings, and still, they were having trouble keeping my oxygen levels up. I routinely attempted to remove the breathing tube, so they had to restrain me. I wasn't sedated, because my blood pressure was so low, so unfortunately, I remember almost the entire stay in the ICU. I remember the respiratory therapist coming in to suction me. It felt like I was being drowned and choked all at the same time. For medical personnel reading this, I beg you not to push the suction so far down the endotracheal tube that it hits the carina (base of the trachea). To this day, it was the most painful thing I have ever experienced.

My vital signs would worsen when my family left, so the ICU broke the rules and allowed someone to be with me 24/7. When they were with me, I would put my hands as together as they could be in restraints, in a prayer-like posture, which was my way of asking them to remove the restraints so I could write. I had a clipboard with paper, and I wrote notes, which I still have today, thanks to my amazing mom. In reality, I just told people what to do, which is super fitting if you know me. I would even ask the respiratory therapist to show me the blood gas results, and then I would write on the paper how I wanted them to wean the settings. Once an ICU nurse, always an ICU nurse.

The doctors had told my family I would be in the ICU for a long time. They said I would likely need a gastrostomy tube (G-tube), which is a tube going into my stomach for feedings, and a tracheostomy for long-term ventilation. Luckily, God had a different plan. I was in the ICU for 7 days, 4 of which were on a ventilator. There is so much I remember from being in the ICU: the ventilator, the monitors, central and arterial lines, the pain, frustration, and a significant lack of control over anything and everything. It was a nightmare I hope I never have to encounter again.

I remember that shortly after the tube was removed, my husband told me that our babies were cremated, and the plan was to keep them with us. He wanted to build a memorial garden at our house and have them there, which I initially disagreed with. However, I eventually warmed up to the idea and loved having them nearby. Later, I found out that they had kept the babies in the morgue at the hospital because they were waiting until I died, and then they would take us all to the funeral home and cremate us together. Even as I write this out, it is hard to fathom.

Once I was transferred out of the ICU, I was placed in a single room (which, at the time, was rare). Folks would come to visit me, and everyone was so happy. You see, everyone had expected that all three of us were going to die, so when I lived, it was a joyous occasion for everyone *except* me. I was devastated. These babies we had worked so hard for were gone. How could it be? To cheer me up, my family snuck in my precious Skeeter Bug. Dogs weren't allowed in the hospital, but she fit perfectly inside a purse, and for a glimpse of a moment, a brief smile returned to my face.

My coworkers from the NICU would come to see me, but I could tell it was hard for them. On the one hand, they were so happy I was alive, and on the other hand, they were so devastated at the loss of the twins we had worked so hard for. They would make small talk, but it was strained, at best. I really just wanted to go home and lock myself in the nursery with Skeeter Bug and cry.

After numerous times begging to be discharged and perhaps even threatening to leave against medical advice (AMA), the MD finally agreed. I got pretty "spicy" toward the end of my stay at the hospital. I was just done. I'm not proud of how I behaved, but I also am compassionate to myself, knowing I was doing the best I could do. You see, often, when people lose all sense of control over their outcomes, they try to control whatever they can. For me, that was attempting to control my care at the hospital; however, there was so much outside of my control. If you are in the healthcare field—or work with people in any capacity—and find yourself dealing with someone who is a bit on the spicy side, I challenge you to be curious. What is going on in that person's life that might be causing them to act the way they are? To quote the famous Ted Lasso, "Be curious, not judgmental."

They eventually put in a peripherally inserted central catheter (PICC) line so I could administer IV antibiotics at home (which I had to do for a month). We picked up the supplies from the home health agency and headed home. I struggled to breathe, but I just wanted to go home. As we arrived home, I went straight to the nursery and opened the door. But what I saw when I opened the door was unexpected. The room was back exactly like before we turned it into a nursery. Apparently, the neighbors had all gotten together and helped to transform the room back into an office. Even the walls were repainted white.

They had taken everything back, and what couldn't be taken back was donated to Good Will. I quickly asked my husband about the plush pink rocking chair, and he told me they had canceled the order. They canceled it. I couldn't believe it. Everything I wanted was gone; at that point, I wished I had just died. At least then I could have been with Joey and Callie—in heaven, where there is no more pain and no more tears. After all, it seemed that here on Earth, the pain and tears would be never-ending.

I walked back to my bedroom and crawled into bed. I called for Skeeter, remembering the feeling of her against my stomach and longing for that feeling again. She quickly jumped in bed (she was more excited about a nap than a walk). She did her routine of three circles by my belly and then walked down by my feet to go to sleep. Words can't really describe how devastating this was. My life shattered into a million pieces and felt like it would never get better.

The days ahead dragged on like pure torture. Friends and family would sometimes come by, but it was awkward at best. We would also see friends out at the grocery stores or other public places and notice they were avoiding us. It was almost as if our grief was a communicable disease they might "catch" if they were to get near us. One of my key takeaways from enduring this tragic situation was that there were never any words that made it better. I would rather someone sit with me and say, "I'm so sorry" and then just be quiet. It is in our nature to fill the silence with words, but in reality, in situations like these, words are just words and often do more harm than good.

The other thing I noticed people would try to do is to "fix" it with statements that started with "Well, at least ..." I learned quickly to ignore anything that came after "Well, at least." People might say things like, "Well, at least you know you can get pregnant," "Well, at least you lived," or "Well, at least you have two angels in Heaven." I knew in my heart that people were not trying to be hurtful by saying these things. They were simply trying to fill the void of silence, but I preferred silence all day long versus the inappropriate comments. Perhaps a key takeaway you might have from reading this story is that it is okay, in fact likely preferred, just to be present with those experiencing an incomprehensible loss. In my opinion, words don't make anything better. It's your connection and presence that truly matters.

Then came the time to plant the memorial garden. I don't remember the unfortunate landscapers hired to do the job, but I still feel sorry for them. Richard and I were supposed to decide on the design and the plants, but I didn't have it in me. Every time we met with the landscapers, they would ask me questions about what I wanted, and I would say something along the lines of, "I want the nursery back. I want my babies back. I don't want this d*** garden." Despite my inappropriate behavior, by the grace of God, they kept coming back. We had rocks engraved with Joey and Callie's names and their footprints. There were numerous plants but only one with pink flowers and one with blue flowers. They were hydrangeas and were situated right behind their engraved rocks, directly above where their ashes were buried.

The memorial garden wasn't what I wanted, and while I initially resisted the garden, it ended up being my favorite place at our home. Sometimes, I would go outside and lie in the garden for hours. Something about being in the garden made me feel closer to Joey and Callie. When we later got our golden retriever, Sammie Sam, she walked out back, and the first place she went was the garden. I freaked out thinking she was going to potty in the garden, but instead, she did a few circles and laid right between their rocks, directly above where they were buried. I want to think that, somehow, she just knew. I know they would have been the best of friends.

The days turned into weeks, and somehow, I kept moving forward. I guess I didn't have another choice. When I went back to the hospital to have the PICC line removed, I remember sitting in the doctor's office and him looking at my chart and saying, "I have no idea how you survived. God must have big plans for you." I reflected on that statement and tried to trust in God's plan, all the while assuming a part of the plan was for us to have another child; after all, we had frozen embryos.

I soon became obsessed with getting pregnant again. My doctor had great caution about me getting pregnant again; however, he knew I wouldn't take no for an answer, so he set up for us to have another embryo implanted. I prayed and prayed and prayed for it to "work" this time, but it didn't. The embryo survived the thaw but not the implant. I wasn't pregnant, and the likelihood of me ever being pregnant was basically impossible. Because of the emergency nature of the D&C, they likely took too many of the basal cells (cells responsible for growing the uterine lining and ultimately being the home for an embryo). So, not only did we lose our twins but we also lost the possibility of ever getting pregnant again. The thought was unfathomable. I questioned God, wondering how He could let this happen to us. We would have been great, loving parents. It just didn't make sense.

As if things couldn't get worse, about a month after being discharged from the hospital, my hair began falling out. I was losing handfuls of hair daily. Luckily, I have very thick hair, but still, it was getting thinner by the day. I talked to my doctor, who said that when patients are in organ failure and undergo severe stress, they tend to lose their hair. He said there was a chance I could lose all my hair, but it would eventually grow back. Great. *E. coli* sepsis had already taken so much from me—and now my hair. If you know me, you know how much I love my hair. God blessed me with beautiful hair and a talent to somehow fix it. I was, after all, voted "Best Hair" in high school. I went to see my hairstylist, and she felt the best option would be to cut my long hair off, which I did *not* want to do but did because

I had no other choice. With each cut she made, I cried harder. She was crying too. It sounds like a trivial thing, but to me, it was just one more thing to add to the overwhelming heartache.

Years later, my hair grew back to the length it previously was. This time, I grew it as long as I could to purposefully cut it for donation. I loved the thought of a little girl having my hair, just like Callie would have. This time when we cut my hair, it was emotional—but for a different reason. Instead of being told I had to do it, I was doing it because I wanted to, which made it much more meaningful.

Referring to the story with Tyler and Kellie Penn (Part III. It Wasn't Supposed to Happen), as I had walked with them through the loss of their son, Miles, they walked alongside us through the loss of Joey and Callie. As time went on, with the constant support of family and friends, God began healing my broken heart. At Joey and Callie's memorial service, we sang the hymn "It Is Well With My Soul." If I had to be honest, it wasn't really "well" with my soul then. I struggled to find anything "well" about the situation besides that I had lived. But here's the thing: At the time I would have been okay not to have lived.

As the weeks turned into months and I became stronger, I was finally able to be released from my medical leave and return to work in the NICU, which I knew would not be easy. My friends welcomed me with open arms and tried to ensure I started with easier assignments. However, on my first day back, I admitted Tyler and Kellie Penn's daughter, Millie (Part V. Not Again!), which was the farthest thing from an "easy" assignment.

One of the more challenging parts of returning was when support staff would ask how my baby was. They assumed I was back from maternity leave. They had no idea the nightmare I had been through, nor did I really want to get into it when I was supposed to be caring for other babies. Many times, the nurses would intercept staff before they got to me, which was incredibly thoughtful, but sometimes, they just couldn't.

I had also enrolled in a clinical study for moms of twins. They planned to follow me through the pregnancy and the first 2 years of the twins' lives. So, the first time they called for an update after the twins died, I told them what had happened and then asked to be taken off the call list. Except, they kept calling. Each time I got a little more irritated, which honestly happened a lot. There were times I had an overwhelming amount of empathy when folks would ask how my twins were doing, and other times I would snap and become someone I didn't know I was capable of being. These definitely were not my proudest moments. But here's the thing: I was doing the best I could.

I also remember going to counseling before I returned because I had no idea what to say when the baby's parents would ask me if I had children. Almost every parent asked me that question, and I knew it would continue. Saying "no" didn't feel right, as I was acting as if Joey and Callie didn't exist. However, saying "yes" was complex, as it was a complicated and private matter and not necessarily professional to share with a family whose baby I was caring for. The counselor and I ultimately came up with the phrase, "Yes, I have twins in Heaven." Once Kevin and I were married, I would say, "I have three stepsons and twins in Heaven." Some folks would ask for more information, but most just nodded and moved on, not knowing what to say.

I didn't go to deliveries for the first year back in the NICU. My friends would pick up the role of the delivery nurse so I didn't have to do it. I knew it would just be too hard, and I had the best coworkers in the world. Fortunately, the hospital I worked at had just built a new tower, which meant our NICU and L&D were getting an entirely new unit and building. This also meant I wouldn't be forced to go into the room I delivered in or the OR I almost died in. Thank goodness.

I vividly remember the first micro preemie delivery I went to after the year was up. It was a 22-week baby, and we were there to do comfort care. The parents were distraught and didn't want to hold the baby. As you will learn in the upcoming stories, I never let a baby die in the bed, so I picked up this precious baby and held them close to my chest. I could feel them breathing their last breath, and memories of holding Joey and Callie came flooding back. I just stood there, frozen, with tears streaming down my face. Luckily, the nurse practitioner could see I was struggling and asked if she could take the baby and hold them so I could step out.

I handed her the baby and left the delivery room. As I left, I was crying uncontrollably. I got to our break room, and thoughts from my own delivery came flooding over me. I began to hyperventilate, and I didn't have a phone to call for help, nor could I get up and get to the phone on the wall. I don't remember who came in, but they found me passed out and called a code "speed," which was not a full code but still got the team to come quickly.

Once I came to, I was so embarrassed. How could I let this happen? I had been to counseling and done all the things. However, grief is a tricky beast. It will hijack you before you even have a chance to understand what is happening, and you never know when it will hit. Elizabeth Kübler-Ross outlined the five stages of grief as denial, anger, bargaining, depression, and acceptance.[1] I used to think the grieving process was linear in fashion, almost as if you could check the boxes in a row and then be done with it. Well, I was definitely wrong. Even 17 years later, I can be right back in any of the stages. There's zero logic to it, and that is okay.

A little over a year after Joey and Callie died, my husband Richard and I separated. We were both on our own unique path of grieving, ultimately leading to our divorce. It was complicated, to say the least. I was able to stay at the house where Joey and Callie were buried, and of course, I kept Skeeter Bug. She was my faithful sidekick for 18 years until she crossed the rainbow bridge. I hope she is playing with Joey and Callie and that we will all be reunited someday.

Being alone was not easy. I honestly had never been alone. Richard and I had started dating when I was in high school. Being with him was all I knew. Having our marriage end shortly after losing the twins was devastating, but little did I know God's amazing plans for my future. I eventually began dating my current husband, Kevin, and about 2 years after the loss of Joey and Callie, we were married. He had three sons who were such a blessing in my life. We had plans to adopt, but after several years of being on an

---

1 Elizabeth Kübler-Ross, *On Death and Dying* (New York: Simon & Schuster, 2011).

adoption list and not being chosen, we removed our names from the list and got a golden retriever, Sammie Sam. Later, we adopted a spunky hunting dog named Jäger (German for "hunter"). The boys are grown, and Sammie crossed the rainbow bridge in 2021. Now all that remains at our lake home is Jäger and us—our own little slice of Heaven.

My entire family celebrates Joey and Callie each year on their Heaven day. When we held their memorial service, each person had one pink and one blue balloon, which we released at the end. We continued this tradition each year on their Heaven day. However, we eventually transitioned to using biodegradable lanterns. Seeing them fly into the night sky is a scene I will always treasure. Once we moved to the lake, we began releasing water lanterns off our dock, each family member having their own to release. We also have breakfast for supper during their Heaven day celebration. Joey and Callie were super active after I ate breakfast, so we joked about how much they loved it, just like their mommy. My nieces and nephew may never have met Joey and Callie, but they definitely know who they were. To this day, we honor that tradition and will continue until I am reunited with them in Heaven.

I have had the unique opportunity to get a second chance at life, and I do not take that lightly. I get to do things I was never supposed to be able to do. I have summited Mt. Whitney, ran half marathons, started an organic personal care product business, hiked the Maroon Bells Four Pass Loop, went on multiple mission trips, started a non-profit for teaching others about health and wellness, became a yoga instructor, and had countless other adventures. Life is a precious gift, and I am so thankful my time here on Earth didn't end in March of 2006. My goal is that God would continue to use my life to be a blessing to others, regardless of my "job." None of us know how long we have on this Earth. One day, I will be reunited with Joey and Callie, but until then, I plan on living this super snazzy life God has blessed me with. Elizabeth Kübler-Ross says, "The most beautiful people we have known are those who have known defeat, known suffering, known struggle, known loss, and have found their way out of those depths."[2] Finding my way "out" was not easy. There are still days I struggle. However, each day, I consciously choose positive over negative, light over darkness, and faith over fear, with the ultimate understanding that it has been and always will be *well* with my soul.

Reflection Questions

1. What stood out to you most about Valerie's personal story?
2. If you were the nurse in the operating room, how might you have advocated for your patient?
3. Putting yourself in Valerie's shoes, do you think you could have returned to work in the NICU? Regardless of your answer, consider why you answered that way (there is no right or wrong answer).
4. How do you think you personally would have handled it when parents in the NICU asked if you had children?
5. Imagine that you are the person calling Valerie from the clinical trial. How would you have handled the phone call when she was polite? How about when her behavior was on the spicy side?
6. Reflect on the final quote in the story by Elizabeth Kübler-Ross about people who have known loss. What within the quote speaks to you, if anything?
7. Is there anything from Valerie's story that you can personally relate to? How does that make you feel?

---

2 Elizabeth Kübler-Ross, *Death: The Final Stage of Growth* (New York: Simon and Schuster, 1997).

PART II

Contributing Author NICU Stories

About the Contributors

Laura Bowgren, BSN, RN, graduated with her BSN in 2005 and went straight to the NICU, where Valerie was her preceptor. Laura continues to work in the NICU, and according to her, she'll "probably never leave."

Kelli Daugherty, MSN, APRN, CNM, has been a nurse since 2004 and has a passion for all aspects of maternal-child healthcare. She became a NICU nurse after her daughter was born prematurely and spent time in the NICU. She worked in the NICU for 7 years before becoming a nurse midwife to have, in her own words, "the best of both worlds." When Kelli isn't delivering a baby, you might find her teaching nursing students as a maternal-child clinical instructor. Kelli loves her job and also loves spending time with her family, especially her new granddaughter.

Jennifer Rigdon, BSN, RN, CRHCP, graduated from nursing school in 2006. She worked as a NICU nurse for 13 years before becoming a specialty manager in an outpatient clinic. Jennifer is one of the many nurses Valerie had the privilege to help orient to the NICU.

Diedra Stewart MSN, CNL, CLC, graduated with her bachelor's degree in nursing in 1992 and her master's degree in nursing (clinical nurse leader specialty) in 2009. She has worked in the NICU for 31 years and is currently the perinatal network administrator at her local Level III NICU. Diedra, affectionately known to her friends and family as DeDe, has been the rock to many, including Valerie, as they navigated through graduate school together.

Linda Jo Swartz, RNC, became a nurse in 1980. She graduated with her associate's degree in nursing after transferring her coursework from the University of Illinois, where she obtained her undergraduate degree in German with a minor in Russian history and a graduate degree in library science. She worked briefly on a medical-surgical floor before moving to her true passion, the NICU, where she worked for almost 40 years. Linda was in the NICU when I started and was one of the nurses who helped with my orientation. Linda recently retired and is enjoying her time with her friends and family and, of course, keeping up with the lives she touched from all her years in the NICU.

Kathey Voelker, RNC, NNP, graduated with her BSN in 1977, became a neonatal nurse in 1979, and then a neonatal nurse practitioner in 1988. She worked for 37 years in the NICU before retiring to spend time with her family, friends, and beloved animals.

Christine Wetzel, DNP, RNC-NICU, IBCLC, became a nurse in 1993. She spent 18 months as a pediatric nurse before transferring to the NICU in 1995. Dr. Wetzel continues to work as a nurse at the bedside in the NICU. She is passionate about the small baby unit and research to improve babies' lives in the NICU. Additionally, she has the privilege of teaching our future generation of nurses as a part-time nursing instructor at the local university where she resides.

Mary Jayne Zonfrilli, NNP-BC, graduated from nursing school in December of 1976 and became a neonatal nurse practitioner in 1982. Her career in the NICU spanned from 1977 to 2020. She is retired and enjoying time with her family and precious granddogs, Mia and Leo.

Time Changes Everything

Christine Wetzel, DNP, RNC-NICU, IBCLC

As a NICU nurse, my days are often filled with meeting the demands of babies who are beginning to feel stronger and match the energy of the louder and stronger full-term babies. There are days I can barely sit because one of my tiny patients seems to have a sensor for the fact that my hands are free and that I most certainly should be meeting their new demand. I often laugh at the tiny, little baby and reach my hands through the isolette to provide some comfort before I can settle into my charting for a few minutes. I adore the babies and am grateful for my opportunity to be their caregiver. I'm actually grinning while writing this because I just finished a 12-hour shift with two babies who kept me busy and also made me laugh during my shift.

Let me tell you about one of the babies. She is still on her healing journey. She was born at 22 weeks and is still progressing toward steps to go home. There have been days that we told the parents she might not last more than a few more hours. She certainly has had a difficult road. But she is alive and getting stronger every day. She no longer has IV lines dripping fluid into her tiny veins. She can have tube feedings of her mother's own milk. She no longer has a breathing tube, and since her tiny cries are no longer stopped by the breathing tube, we can hear her precious voice. To listen to her cry is like hearing angels sing because there were dark days when we believed that she would not be able to survive. This blessed baby is God's miracle, and through Him, we have advanced our care, treatments, and protocols so that a tiny 22-week baby might not have certain death but instead have a chance to live. We rejoice with the family and marvel at her because she lives.

The painful part is that many infants still lose their lives to prematurity. Prematurity is a leading cause of death in the United States, but a sadder fact is that there are babies who are never even given a chance to live because they are considered too young to save. As we advance our care to attempt to save these extremely tiny babies, I marvel at their size. These babies are so small that their blood pressure cuffs are the size of Band-Aids. They are so tiny that the IV bag dripping lifesaving fluids into their tiny vein weighs more than the baby. They are impossibly small but have the heart of a lion and a will to live as hard as steel. They are so feisty; they even kick me with their tiny feet the size of Trident gum when I change their diapers. It is these babies who make me think of a day many, many years ago when my dear friend and coworker Valerie (the author of this book) was told that her 22-week twins must be delivered and could not be saved.

Valerie tells the story of her twins, but there is so much more to tell you about Valerie and how she was born to be a mother. Valerie was the most adorable pregnant person you could ever meet. She absolutely adored working with the babies in the NICU and is a truly amazing nurse. She made me laugh because every baby she was assigned was given lavish amounts of loving attention. She was ridiculously happy while giving each baby both lifesaving and loving, gentle care.

Valerie sparkled, and her beautiful soul shined more than the bows and ribbons she wore in her gorgeous hair. Her assigned babies had bows in their hair or some cute adornment practically the minute they were out of the womb. You see, Valerie knew how precious the babies were to their families, and she wanted every minute to count. She worked hard to ensure the families had as many warm memories as possible in case the baby did not survive.

I learned from Valerie that families needed memories that make them smile so if hard days came, they would have hope, and if the worst day came and their precious baby was not able to stay in this world, they would have conversations, pictures, footprints, bows, and love to keep in their hearts. If you could see Valerie with a baby, you would know what I know: that she was born to be a mother. So, we were so excited when Valerie got pregnant with the twins. We would, of course, have an extravagant, super snazzy (Valerie's favorite word) baby shower, and I would help her breastfeed because breastfeeding is my unique talent. We (the other NICU nurses) knew that the twins might come early, so we would be ready to be the best nurses for her babies. We could picture Valerie being the best momma, and we were happy to watch her body grow the babies. But sadly, that is not how this story ends. We didn't have that extravagant baby shower, nor did we get to hold and care for her babies.

Instead, we were terrified that Valerie would not only lose the twins, but we would also lose Valerie herself. I don't remember the details, but I remember that Valerie fought to keep those babies alive. All those years ago, 24 weeks was the cutoff to be admitted to NICU. Babies born earlier than 24 weeks were given to the mother and father (or whoever was in the delivery room supporting the mother) and held until they took their last breath. Most survived only minutes. Valerie knew the fate of her twins if they were born before 24 weeks, and she did everything she could to keep those babies inside her womb. You see, Valerie was born to be a mother—a mother who fought for the lives of her babies.

It was a blur of events that were hard to take in. NICU nurses are on this Earth to save babies, and we wanted to save Valerie's babies. We wept when we realized their birth would occur and they could not be saved. We wept when we understood that Valerie had tried so hard to keep the babies in her womb, to give them as much time as possible so that they would survive, that she almost lost her life. Valerie nearly died as her babies, Joey and Callie, were born. As Joey and Callie took their first and ultimately their last breath, Valerie, too, was seemingly taking one of her last breaths.

By the grace of God, Valerie survived. I'm sure Valerie's soul and the twins' souls mingled together in those moments, and those babies felt her strong, beautiful love as Jesus wrapped them in His arms and pushed Valerie back to Earth. You see, Valerie was meant to be a mother, and a mother she is, of two precious angels. I know my friend Valerie waits for that glorious day to feel them in her arms again. But until that day, we get to watch her life continue to unfold. We are so thankful Valerie survived and ultimately returned and worked in our NICU, where she continued to give the same lavishly loving life-saving care. Now that she has transitioned into teaching, I am confident that her students receive the same care and attention. It's just who Valerie is, and I am beyond thankful she survived and can share her stories with this book.

Reflection Questions

1. How do you think having a coworker relationship with a patient would impact your experience treating them? Would it make your job harder or easier?
2. What images or details stand out to you from this story?
3. After reflecting on this story and Valerie's personal story, list three emotions that come up, and why.
4. Although the subject matter is generally sad, what are three positive things that occurred in this story?

Healing Hearts

Christine Wetzel, DNP, RNC-NICU, IBCLC

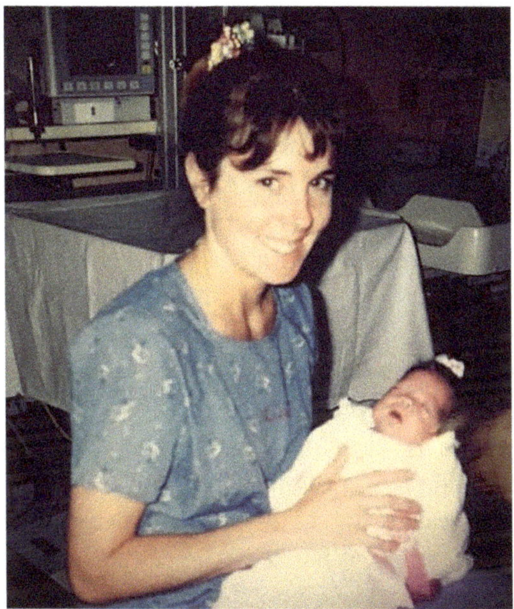

IMG 2.1

The number of families affected by prematurity is staggering. In the United States, about 10% of infants are born prematurely. Globally, approximately 1 million children die every year due to complications of prematurity, making prematurity the leading cause of death in children under 5 years.[1] As a nurse,

1 World Health Organization, "Preterm Birth," May 10, 2023, https://www.who.int/news-room/fact-sheets/detail/preterm-birth.

when I read statistics about premature births, my mind doesn't think about numbers. Every number is a baby—and maybe a baby that was in my unit, in my care. I take these numbers personally.

The reality is that most premature babies fall into the category of "late preterm infants," and most do not require admission to the NICU. Most babies aren't admitted to the NICU unless they are less than 35 weeks gestation, which would be a little more than a month early. I tell you this to give you a picture of babies of all sizes, with so many reasons that they needed the extra attention of a NICU. Most babies admitted to the NICU stay less than 2 weeks and are happily sent home to their families.

But sometimes something so unexpected and unspeakable happens that there is a tragic turn of events, and a baby is born early, sick, or even injured because a pregnant mother becomes gravely ill or injured herself. NICU nurses are witnesses to very rare events—events that are sometimes shocking, like the mother being a victim of violence, a car accident, a drug overdose, or an illness beyond medical healing. The births of babies in any other of these mentioned circumstances are dire. And the surviving family members are left shocked and at a loss for what to do next. Saying goodbye to their daughter, wife, or girlfriend while expecting a new life is something I was not prepared for as a NICU nurse.

Infant death is a rare event. Maternal death (when the pregnant person dies) is even rarer. When a mother dies, I have found that infant grief is real. Infant grief is not discussed in textbooks or any class I have attended. I'm not sure there is any mention of infant grief in the literature. But I have seen infant grief, and it's heartbreaking. These babies, who lost their mother, need more than just the exceptional medical care that the NICU provides.

We must give pieces of ourselves to the babies and surviving family so that the baby can heal and reach wellness. Tragic events don't trigger a shutdown in most nurses; instead, we go deeper. I recently watched *Thor: Love and Thunder*, and when Jane says to Thor, "Keep your heart open," I felt that. We are taught that nursing is both a science and an art, but the art piece is what I feel in my heart and how I touch and care for a baby. In moments of great sadness, I draw strength from God. As a nurse, I must keep my light burning so I can be the light for the family during their time of darkness and especially so that the infant who has experienced loss can recover.

One baby who experienced the loss of her mother is still a part of my life. She is now an adult with children of her own, but she is still drawn to me after all these years. The love I poured into her while she was in the NICU remains in her heart. Our story is public, and we have been on a few news stories together. But I am going to share with you one of my favorite phone calls in my history of phone calls.

The story goes like this. The baby's name is Christine, and one day she called me to tell me that she had begun dating a nice young man. The tone of her voice made me pause, and I thought to myself, "Gosh, this sounds serious." So, I told her that I would like to meet the young man. She giggled, and she said, "You already know him." I was shocked to think I could know someone she would meet and begin dating, and I waited for her to say more. She told me I knew him because I had also cared for him when he was a baby in the NICU!

Imagine my surprise. Two of my NICU babies met and found a connection with each other! We arranged a get-together, and I could see the love. He totally understood her deepest wounds. This young relationship continued to develop, and I attended their wedding. A beautiful story came from a traumatic birth and difficult NICU stays for both families. I like to think I had a role in their little NICU hearts finding each other.

Reflection Questions

1. Did the number of premature deaths surprise you, or did you think the total was more or less than approximately 1 million annually?
2. How did you feel when you read that two of the babies Chris had cared for ultimately ended up getting married? (When talking to Chris about this story, she revealed that even though she had cared for both babies, they were, in fact, not in the NICU at the same time—close, but not at the same time. What are the chances?)

The Miracle of Birth

Christine Wetzel, DNP, RNC-NICU, IBCLC

My nursing career in the NICU has been filled with breathtaking moments. The progression of our ability to care for babies that were once thought to be too small or too premature to save has been remarkable. When I started in the NICU in 1995, my hospital was cutting edge with admitting 24-week gestation infants. A full-term pregnancy is defined as 37–40 weeks gestation. So a 24-week infant born 4 months early is extremely premature and needs help with everything, including breathing, digesting food, staying warm, coping with the new environment of the NICU, brain development, family support, and on and on and on. Our science has advanced so much over the years that it is now possible to save babies born at 22 weeks gestation!

I am blessed to work in a NICU that attempts to save infants as young as 22 weeks gestation. Many hospitals in the United States have guidelines in place that do not include admitting an infant less than 24 weeks gestation. As a matter of fact, there is a Facebook group named "TwentyTwo Matters" that provides information on which hospitals in the United States are known to attempt to save these extremely premature infants. It has been my experience that these tiny 22- to 23-week infants are fighters, and they are worth our time and effort.

As a team, we practice and study the science of the very best treatments to give these tiny infants a chance at life. First, the parents must understand their choices and the infant's chances of survival. The NICU doctor, who is called a neonatologist, ideally provides counseling to the expectant family. This is where my story about a tiny life starts.

An expectant mother was admitted to the L&D department due to pregnancy complications. Her doctor told her that it was unlikely her baby would survive. The parents desperately wanted this baby and stated they wanted everything done to save their tiny precious baby. While the decisions are being made in the L&D department, the NICU staff is immediately put on alert. What no parent can comprehend at the moment they say they want everything done is that the NICU becomes a hive of activity. We have teams in place, protocols, and standards that are based on the best science, and we propel them into action. The NICU delivery team is a highly specialized team that only appears in deliveries if the infant is at risk for complications. It is this team that will attend the delivery and "help" the baby transition to the NICU world. I am a member of this team. I am privileged to begin the lifesaving steps this impossibly tiny baby will need.

This tiny, extremely premature baby who only weighs about 500 grams (1.1 lbs) is absolutely dependent on our first steps. For a comparison, think about a trauma scene or a severe heart attack victim. Think about what you have seen in a movie or witnessed yourself. Life hangs in the balance in these extreme cases, and specialized equipment along with registered nurses, neonatologists, neonatal nurse practitioners (NNP), and respiratory therapists enter the delivery room to focus on the baby who is about to be born.

In this case, the parents had been told that it was unlikely that their tiny, extremely premature infant would make it out of the delivery room alive. I can't imagine giving birth and losing your infant within minutes. How do you say hello and goodbye at the same time?

As our NICU team gathered with our equipment and entered into the delivery room, we understood the gravity of the situation. The obstetrician (OB) delivered the baby, and I held my breath waiting to see the baby. My mind raced through the sequence of neonatal resuscitation (NRP), and I prayed that we would be successful at saving this infant. I started the timer the second the baby was born and waited with the isolette open and the heat turned on so that the baby would have the comfort of warmth and the science of thermoregulation immediately ready. I was straining my neck to catch a glimpse of the infant. The OB handed the baby to the NNP, and she gently scooped up the tiny baby. My own heart was racing because I was unable to get a visual of the infant.

For reference, I almost always can catch a glance at the baby during the handoff from OB to NNP. I use those split seconds to assess how vigorous the baby is. Are they moving? Are they attempting to cry? But this baby was so impossibly tiny that I could not see the baby at all. Those 2 seconds might have been the longest seconds of my life. I was most likely holding my breath.

The NNP stepped to the head of the opened isolette, lowered her closed hands, and slowly and gently opened her hands to reveal one of the tiniest babies I had ever seen. I quickly began the steps of NRP, and we all began to smile as we watched this impossibly small baby begin to breathe, turn pink, and kick his tiny feet. You could compare his feet with a piece of Trident gum. This baby was a miracle. We quickly called the infant's father to come to look at his tiny perfect infant, who was very much alive. We celebrated with the dad and mom for about 10 seconds or less and quickly took the baby to the NICU.

In the NICU, we took this baby to a specialized area called the small baby unit (SBU). The SBU nurses have extra training and experience and were hopefully waiting for the unlikely event that we would be bringing a new baby into the SBU. I couldn't stop smiling. The delivery team transferred care to the SBU team, and I stood with the infant's father. Together, we marveled at the sight of his beautiful tiny baby. His emotions could not be contained. He sunk to his knees in gratitude and could no longer stop the tears from flowing. He tried to explain his tears, but now I was crying with him, and he looked at me and realized he didn't need to explain at all. Miracles don't need explanations.

Reflection Questions

1. What are your thoughts about the technology of healthcare advancing so that 22-week babies could be saved?
2. What ethical principles do you think come into play when resuscitating 22-week infants?
3. What do you think it would be like to work as a NICU nurse in the SBU?
4. Imagine yourself for a moment as a nurse in the SBU. What emotions would you have felt seeing the father from this story fall to his knees?

The Power of Warmth

Kathey Voelker, RNC, NNP

It was a cold and snowy Saturday. My attending and I had just finished rounds and reviewed what we'd done when a call came in from the emergency department (ED). The 911 dispatch had notified them of an anonymous call they had received from a young woman who told the 911 operator that she had given birth and had left the baby in a cemetery under the pine trees. The police and the fire departments had started the search, and the baby would be brought to us if it was found in time.

We started setting up what we needed. We got a temperature-controlled heating pad for under the baby, a bear-hugger (a paper tube that surrounds the baby with warm air) we had used in the OR, a heater used to warm IV fluids, and, of course, full resuscitation equipment.

There are three cemeteries in town. Worried that there were not enough people looking, an off-duty fireman headed out to search. He was the one who found her, just as described, in a blanket under a tree. She was brought immediately to us for resuscitation and care.

Amazingly, she was responsive, although minimally. Her temperature was too low to register. We applied all the resources we had and slowly, safely warmed her up. Once warm, she woke up, cried, and responded to touch and sound. This was before the practice of cooling the brain in cases of asphyxia, but our guess is it worked the same way because she started acting like a regular newborn. Over the next few weeks, she grew and gained weight. A foster family was found for her, and she was discharged without incident.

Fast forward 15 years later. I was teaching a class on stabilization for transport at a community hospital, and I was talking about the importance of safe warming. I told this story to emphasize the importance of warming. After the talk, a woman approached me and said, "I was the one that adopted her. She's a completely normal teenager. Would you like to meet her?" Well, of course I did! I was thrilled. She picked her up from the high school and brought her to meet me. I would never have imagined I'd have the opportunity to see this "baby" again after all these years. Today, she is a beautiful, intelligent young woman, and I am grateful to have had the closure of meeting her—but this time under different and much happier circumstances.

Reflection Questions

1. What emotions came up when you read that the baby's mother left her in a cemetery on a cold winter day? Why do you think you felt those emotions? As a practice of empathy, list several possible reasons a mother could find herself in this situation.
2. Put yourself in Kathey's shoes. What might it have felt like getting to meet this miracle "baby" now as an adult?
3. After reviewing the resources provided at the end of this book, what do you think the chances of survival were of the baby in this story?

Defying the Odds

Kelli Daugherty, MSN, APRN, CNM

I never pictured myself being a NICU nurse until my daughter was born prematurely, and suddenly, I found myself engulfed in infant IVs, tube feedings, phototherapy, and respiratory support. And then I knew that as a nurse, I could bring legitimate empathy to those other parents and care for their babies in the way I wanted my own baby cared for. After 7 years of being a NICU nurse, I have countless stories and experiences, but there is one baby that I can't forget.

This sweet baby was born at 32 weeks and eventually developed bronchopulmonary dysplasia. He spent several months in the NICU with a tracheostomy and on a ventilator. He coded a lot. At least two or three times per week. Every time our team was on their game, he would be resuscitated quickly. If I were caring for him that night, I would call his mom, and it would break my heart to have to tell her that it was happening again. My fear was always that there would come a day when he would no longer be able to be resuscitated and I would have to make a very different phone call.

And one night, I thought that was it. He coded, and it took multiple rounds of chest compressions and medications this time, not just one. In what was probably only 15 minutes, my mind felt like it took hours to get him back. I thought that was the beginning of the end for him. After the rest of the team dispersed, I was alone at his bedside. I walked over to his crib and looked at him. He looked back at me with a look that I can only describe as sadness—just big, sad eyes. I stroked his little head full of dark hair and said, "I know, Buddy. You were just up there having coffee with Jesus, and we brought you back again. It's not very nice. I'm sorry." I watched as he scrunched his little face up, as if he understood what I was saying, and a single tear fell out of his eye.

As time went on, the routine continued until he was stable. He quit coding and didn't need resuscitating regularly. Then never. Eventually, he got to go home! He did go home with his tracheostomy and ventilator, but he was home! It was not a day I expected would ever happen. I thought of him on occasion over the years and wondered how he was. Was he still alive? Did he ever get off the ventilator? NICU nurses see hundreds of babies and don't always get updates. One day, several years later, I was out shopping and recognized the baby's father at a store. He moved, and I realized that walking behind him was a little boy with a head full of dark hair and a healed tracheostomy scar on his neck. I silently thanked God for the update I'd been longing for.

Reflection Questions

1. Kelli became a NICU nurse after having a NICU experience of her own. How do you think her experience helps her care for these babies and comfort the parents?
2. The baby in this story required chest compressions two or three times a week, meaning he was near death multiple times a week. What effect do you think this would have on you as a NICU nurse?
3. Kelli mentions the fact that NICU nurses rarely get updates on the patients they helped care for, but she did recognize the baby in the story several years later while out shopping. She doesn't mention whether she reached out or said hi to the boy and his father. Would you have tried to make contact? Why, or why not?

The Longest Transport

Mary Jayne Zonfrilli, NNP-BC

In my early NICU years and until the early 2000s, we had no designated transport team at the hospital I worked at. A registered nurse (RN) and a respiratory therapist (RT) went on transports, and later a neonatal nurse practitioner (NNP) was added to that team. The RN who went was usually whoever was the least busy at the time the call came in.

A particularly complicated transport occurred one summer day. We received a call from a small hospital in our region approximately 2 hours away by ambulance. Our team set out to pick up an infant with respiratory distress. The RN who was chosen to go preferred low-risk infants, or what we so lovingly called "feeders and growers," but she was the least busy, so off we went.

As we arrived, the referring hospital's pediatrician, nurses, and respiratory therapist were conducting full resuscitation on the infant, whose condition had deteriorated while we were en route. Our team jumped into action and led the resuscitative efforts with our collaborating NICU doctor on the phone for guidance. The infant required constant resuscitation, antibiotics, blood gases, X-rays, and blood transfusions to stabilize for transfer. The transport RN performed skillfully in her duties with the infant.

At this particular time in my life, I had just learned I was pregnant and hadn't shared the news with anyone at work. In this stressful situation, I began feeling lightheaded from not eating for several hours. I let the newborn nursery staff know what was going on. They immediately sat me down, gave me juice, and made me a sandwich. During this time, the pediatrician continued caring for the infant.

We stayed at the referring hospital for four hours, making every attempt at stabilization. Our NICU doctor then gave us the okay to begin our transport back. We resuscitated the infant the entire way back. Unfortunately, the infant was diagnosed with overwhelming sepsis at the end of this 8-hour transport. Despite our efforts, he passed away a few hours after our return.

Upon reviewing our experience, our team collaborated well with the referring hospital's team and each other. I witnessed outstanding work and rising to the occasion from an RN who otherwise liked to stay on the sidelines, and I couldn't have been prouder of her. I felt love and concern from fellow nurses I didn't know before that day. A few days following this transport, I received a letter of commendation praising myself and my coworkers on our critical thinking, skill, and collaboration during the crucial course of events. Teamwork, after all, is what NICU is all about!

Reflection Questions

1. The NICU nurse in this story spent over 8 hours trying to save this baby. Do you think this extra level of effort made the loss more difficult? If so, why?
2. The story mentions an RN who preferred to work with low-risk infants, referred to as “feeders and growers.” Do you think you would prefer to work with low-risk or high-risk infants? Why?
3. Think back to a time when you were involved with a team and the outcome was not as you had planned. How did you handle the challenge and, ultimately, the defeat?

A Christmas Miracle

Linda Jo Swartz, RNC

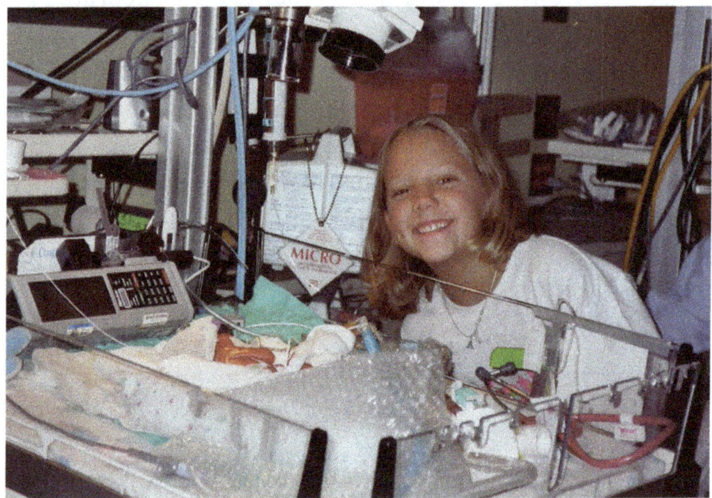

IMG 2.2

In my years at the NICU, I almost always worked the Christmas Eve shift so I could have Christmas Day off. And so it was that 20 years ago I was working a Christmas Eve shift. Back then, we only had three or four nurses working per shift. That year, we had a 25-week infant named Zachary whose family visited often, and Christmas Eve was no exception. However, this day was different.

We got a call that the parents and their daughter had been in a car accident. Everyone was okay, but they would have to stay in our rooming-out room because their car was totaled and they couldn't get a replacement on Christmas Eve. Their young daughter Ana was distraught that Santa wouldn't be able to find her and she wouldn't have any Christmas.

When we learned that Ana was so worried, we three nurses went into action. We called our homes and families, including our children, asking all of them to think about things they could give Ana. Someone came up with a small Christmas tree. My daughter gave me one of her precious dolls. Families brought wrapping paper, special treats, and other toys for Ana. We wrapped presents between caring for our patients and had it all set up for Ana in the morning. The family was overwhelmed, and Ana was ecstatic. The three NICU nurses working that night had truly pulled off a "Christmas miracle."

I cared for this family for many days before Zachary was finally discharged. I taught the mother how to give her fragile baby boy a bath. When she was afraid, I encouraged her. At one of our annual reunions years later, with tears in her eyes, Ana's mother, Tammy, told me how much I meant to her. I was the first nurse that taught her how to give her delicate premature baby a bath. I was also one of the nurses that helped to orchestrate a Christmas miracle that, even to this day, Ana still remembers. Tammy was overwhelmingly grateful for all I had done for her entire family.

You see, being a nurse to me meant far more than "just" providing medical care to my patients.

I had a special bond with this family that extended far beyond their time in the NICU. I attended the baby's baptism and kept up with the family until they moved to Hawaii.

Years later, a man came to our house to fix our phone. He saw my license plate that read "NEORN," asked who I was, and then told me how I had cared for his son, Zachary. Little did I know they had moved back to Illinois! Fast forward to 2019. My mother fell and was admitted to the hospital. The following week when she was receiving physical therapy, the student therapist was none other than Ana! God has sustained the Christmas miracle by continuing to weave our lives together, and for that, I am incredibly grateful.

Reflection Questions

1. The nurses in this story went out of their way to make the holiday special for Ana, the patient's sister. Do you think this went "above and beyond" their duties as NICU nurses? Would you have done the same?
2. Have you encountered a similar situation where your life path continued to weave into another life in coincidental and seemingly miraculous ways? If so, how did it make you feel?

Open Heart and Home

Linda Jo Swartz, RNC

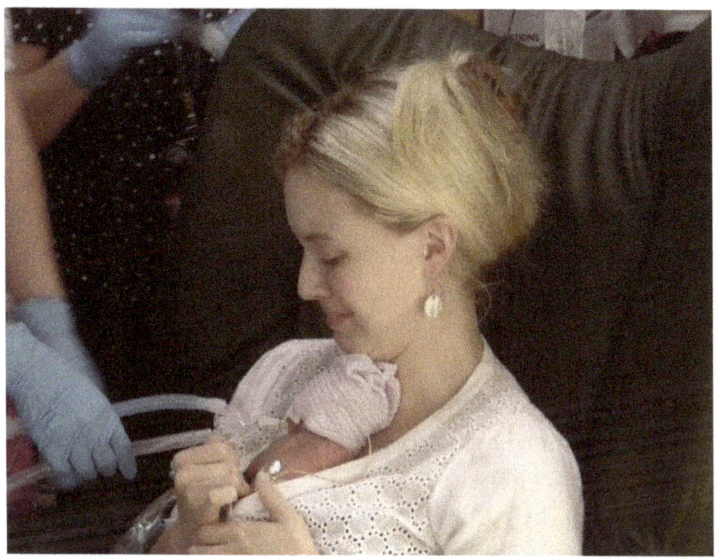

IMG 2.3

Kendra (a 24-week baby girl) wasn't my patient, but I was asked to sit by her bedside while her nurse was at lunch. As I arrived at her bedside, I noticed her mom, Melissa, was crying. I pulled my chair closer, laid a hand on Melissa's shoulder, and asked, "Do you want to tell me what's bothering you?" It was as if you could physically see the relief in her body as her story poured out from her heart.

Melissa had come to Illinois from Oregon to take a review class for her boards for her doctor of medicine. While in Illinois, she went into labor at 24 weeks. A fellow student took her to our hospital to get checked out, and shortly after that, she delivered. She could stay in our hospital's guest house for 2 weeks, and they extended it for 2 more but couldn't let her stay longer. Then, somehow, she was connected to a family needing a house sitter for a while. At the time, I was sitting by her bedside, that family was returning, and she didn't know what she was going to do.

I was struck by the similarity of her situation to my own daughter living in Texas, who was due on almost the same date in September, and I couldn't imagine her being in a place so far from home and not having any place to stay close to her baby. I felt compelled to help. I told Melissa that I needed to speak to my husband to be sure but that I felt confident we could let her stay in our basement finished room. He agreed immediately, and Melissa moved in with us soon after that. I didn't tell anyone at the hospital what we were doing, as I was concerned they would feel I had "gone too far" with this family. As nurses, we aren't supposed to "get too attached," but God had different plans. Honestly, I have zero regrets and would do the same thing all over if I had the chance.

In all, she was with us until Kendra's discharge in September, about 8 weeks. When we were getting ready to go to Texas for my daughter's delivery, Melissa's mother and grandparents drove cross country, bringing their RV to bring Kendra and Melissa home. We invited them to stay at our house until Kendra's discharge day, saying that it was silly to pay for a hotel when we had plenty of beds.

Becky, Melissa's mom, asked my husband before we left, "Why would you do this for us? You don't know us!" And my husband replied, "God tells us to care for our neighbor, and even though we didn't know you, you are still our neighbor." (Love your neighbor as yourself—Lev. 19:18) If I hadn't been asked to sit by Kendra's bedside that day, I wouldn't have known her story or her need. I truly believe that God brings people into our lives for a reason. To this day, I am still in contact with Melissa and her family. While my husband and I opened our home to this family, I believe it truly was God who opened our hearts and, ultimately, our home for this family in need.

When reaching out to Melissa for permission to use their names in this story, she sent the following reply:

We are forever grateful and in debt of the kindness of strangers, especially to Linda and her husband Bruce for giving me a place to live while Kendra was in the hospital. I stayed in Illinois for the ~5 months that Kendra was in the NICU. We had no money, so I have no idea what we would have done without Linda and Bruce. It was so nice to have a safe place to go to when I left the hospital each night.

Reflection Questions

1. What is your reaction to Linda inviting this family to stay at her home? Do you think it is appropriate in certain cases for nurses to be involved with patients and/or their families outside of the hospital setting?
2. Linda said Melissa's situation made her think of her own daughter. Do you think this may have influenced her desire to extend special help to her? Why else do you think nurses might get attached to some patients and their families more than others?
3. Linda mentions that nurses are generally instructed not to "get too attached" to their patients. Why do you think this is? Do you agree or disagree? Explain your answer.

The Nosebleed Miracle

Laura Bowgren, BSN, RN

In the main operating room (OR), a mother, 7 months pregnant with twins, was having a routine surgery on her nose to help to stop her nosebleed. The surgeon said, "Nothing will happen, but let's play it safe and have a NICU nurse there." This seemingly offhand decision turned out to be a matter of life and death.

As the backup delivery nurse, I received a frantic call: "They're crashing, the twins in the main OR. I need more hands now!" I ran the short distance from the NICU with extra equipment in hand and more help trailing shortly behind. When I emerged through the doors, I saw the babies lying with a team of people over them on the warmers, and my mind kicked into high gear as I began caring for Liam.

This sweet, tiny boy didn't seem to be coming around with routine intervention, but we pressed forward. I began chest compressions as a coworker prepared umbilical lines, and another drew up epinephrine to help his tiny heart work without my compressions. My mind was swirling amidst the chaos to be sure we were working together. You see, running a code is like a structured dance for us as we verbalize the help needed, all the while thinking about the next intervention.

Once Liam was intubated, had his umbilical lines attached, and his heart was beating independently, he was stable enough to transport to the NICU for further care and interventions. During the admission, we noticed he started to have seizure-like movements, and my heart sank. Given the intensity of interventions needed for him in the first moments of life,

I grappled with knowing a brain bleed was a possibility, and these moments were not an encouraging sign.

Within a couple of hours, the mom was stabilized and able to visit her babies for the first time. With her husband at her side, I will never forget her breaking into "Jesus Loves Me." It broke my heart and made me smile simultaneously. That night I left work feeling incredibly heavy, sad, and with dwindling hope that Liam would still be there when I returned a couple of days later.

In the coming weeks, Lian and Noah both improved, and their initial head ultrasounds were done. Noah's results were completely normal; however, Liam's report confirmed our fears of severe intraventricular hemorrhage (IVH). This devastating information was shared with the family, and the potential for a long road ahead for him was made clear. We prayed together on many occasions over the boys, and the family continued to make sure the boys knew Jesus loved them both very much.

A repeat head ultrasound was done, and not one of us could have predicted the results; in fact, many staff were in disbelief. It was suggested that the results were switched with his brother, Noah, who previously had a completely normal head ultrasound. Despite all odds, it was true: Miraculously, Liam's grade 3 bleed had completely resolved with no evidence it had ever even existed.

There is no good medical explanation for this, a true miracle I continue to reflect on a decade later as I have the blessing of continuing to watch Liam and Noah grow and thrive! A nosebleed truly was the start of a precious miracle that continues to amaze me 10 years later!

Reflection Questions

1. What do you think would have happened to Liam and Noah had the surgeon not "played it safe" by bringing a NICU nurse in for the routine surgery?
2. What did you think when you read that Liam's grade 3 head bleed had resolved entirely? Is this a normal occurrence for babies in the NICU?

A Single Shift's Tragedy

Jennifer Rigdon, BSN, RN, CRHCP

No one is ever prepared when a baby in the NICU does not live. As nurses, we study and learn all we can to help prevent that from happening, but when it does, it is something you never forget. It has been 7 years, but I still vividly remember caring for a precious baby girl named Gracie (name changed for privacy), who unfortunately did not make it.

I knew her story from my nights as a charge nurse, getting reports on every infant in the unit, but I had never taken care of her before or met her parents. I knew their names, they were sweet people, and they, unfortunately, had a heartbreaking past, as their first baby had died from genetic abnormalities. After so much grief, Gracie was truly a gift, and her parents couldn't wait to take her home.

The night I took care of her for the first time, she moved to a crib during the day, a huge milestone for a NICU baby. Her parents came in to do her 8:00 p.m. feeding and care. We casually chatted as I completed her assessment and they changed her and fed her. She looked good. Her feeding went well. Everything was fine as her parents tucked her into bed after her feeding. I told them I would take good care of her and let them know if there were any changes as I wished them a good night on their way out of the NICU.

At 11:00 p.m., I changed her diaper and did her feeding with no issues. Nothing was amiss as I swaddled her back up after the feeding and laid her back in her crib. In the NICU, we are typically assigned three to four babies, and they eat every 3 hours, so after caring for Gracie, I moved on to care for my other patients who had 11:00 p.m. and midnight feedings. Gracie was sound asleep and hooked up to her monitor, which continuously measured her heart rate and oxygen levels. Her heart rate and oxygen were in the target range as I cared for my other patients and then sat down to complete some charting.

Just after midnight, while charting on my patients, I heard Gracie let out a little whimper: no crying, just a little, soft sound followed by silence as she stayed asleep. About 10 minutes later, she caught my attention again as she let out another little whimper. Still, she stayed sleeping, and her monitor vitals were normal as I continued to finish charting. At 12:45 a.m., Gracie whimpered again. At this point, I decided to check on her early. You see, it is important to let the babies rest between feedings, so we do everything we can not to disturb them between feedings.

When I unswaddled her to check her diaper, she was cold—too cold. I immediately called for a coworker to get me a warmer to lay her on and began doing an assessment. A flurry of activity followed to get her on the warmer so that we could get her body temperature up to normal. Sick babies cannot keep their temperatures up, and this baby was ill. The minute she was placed on the warmer, her oxygen levels started dropping. I called for respiratory therapy, who put her on bubble CPAP (continuous positive airway pressure) to assist with her oxygenation. Bubble CPAP is a noninvasive form of assisting ventilation in newborns with respiratory distress. The baby is doing all the breathing on their own, but the CPAP helps to maintain their lung volume and also provides them with additional oxygen, as needed. Meanwhile, the charge nurse called for the provider to come to the bedside. I could only overhear the charge nurse part of the conversation, but I remember saying to her, "I need the provider up here right now!"

What seemed like only seconds after respiratory therapy put the CPAP on her, she started having apneas that required her to be intubated immediately. Another staff member and I worked to get IV placement in two places and labs drawn, which is routine when we suspect a baby is sick. Shortly after, Gracie's heart rate dropped, and she required CPR. I started chest compressions on her, following the neonatal resuscitation guidelines. I was on autopilot as my mind was in complete disbelief and shock; Gracie was just fine a few hours ago. The parents had been called and rushed back to the NICU. I can still see the look of shock on their faces as tears streamed from their eyes as they took in the scene in front of them.

We did multiple rounds of compressions with epinephrine. Typically, we trade out the role of doing chest compressions, but I refused to let anyone step in to relieve me. Compressions were all I could do during those minutes that seemed to stretch on for hours as her parents looked on in horror and grief at the scene before them. I would not give up doing compressions and trying to save her. I could not leave her bedside to go to her parents after I had told them before they left the unit that I would take good care of their baby. In hindsight, I know I took good care of Gracie, but this time, it just wasn't enough.

Gracie died. Nothing we did, no training we had, could save her. I would later find out that she had a heart defect that was not seen in her routine echocardiogram. I remind myself that we did everything we could. I got in to care for her over an hour earlier than usual because I wanted to ensure she was comfortable. My colleagues that night were quick to get everything done for her. We started CPR immediately when it was needed. We all worked tirelessly and seamlessly to save Gracie. None of that was enough. Gracie's parents were holding her and looking forward to taking her home soon during the beginning of my shift, and by the end of my shift, I was handing these two sweet, kind people their deceased baby girl. Nothing prepares you for that, and it haunts me to this day.

Any one of us could have been in Jennifer's shoes that night. Jennifer is one of the best NICU nurses out there, and I hope that by writing out Gracie's story, she can come to forgive herself, as she did everything humanly possible for sweet Gracie. ~Valerie

Reflection Questions

1. Jennifer seemed to feel extra responsibility for this baby once things took a turn for the worse. Why do you think that is?
2. For NICU nurses, losing a patient can be a haunting and emotional experience. How would you prepare yourself for this reality? What are some sources of strength and comfort you could rely on in this situation?
3. Have you ever second-guessed yourself or felt guilty about something you had no control over? Reflect on the situation and be curious about why you had those feelings. No judgment. Just curious.

From Nurse to Family

Diedra Stewart, MSN, CNL, CLC

Sometimes, things happen for a reason, but we have no idea at the time. As a charge nurse in our NICU, I never was able to be a primary care nurse. I seemed to always be in charge. I attended a delivery of a 32-week infant and brought her to the NICU per protocol. I had no idea the impact this encounter would have on my life. On the rare shift that I was not in charge of, I always seemed to be assigned to care for Kayla. She took her time gaining weight and seemed to hang out in our NICU longer than needed. Looking back, I think that was her way of bringing her mother and me together as friends. The day came for Kayla's discharge, and I knew we would always keep in touch. Well, I was right. Almost 31 years later, I am still a part of her life. Kayla's mom had this wild idea to set me up on a blind date with her husband's cousin. I had no desire to go on a blind date but finally relented and said I would. We did go on our blind date and will be married 29 years this June. Little did I know that my care of Kayla in the NICU would lead me to meet my future husband. God works in mysterious ways.

Reflection Questions

1. Diedra says that things happen for a reason and believes that fate/God brought her and her husband together. Do you agree, or do you tend to believe more in coincidences?

2. There are many stories in this book where the NICU nurses' personal lives were changed because of the care they provided to a baby in the NICU. Why do you think this is? What are some possible advantages and disadvantages to getting involved in patients' and their families' lives?

An Unforgettable Career

Diedra Stewart, MSN, CNL, CLC

It seems like yesterday that I was a new nurse starting my dream career in a Level III NICU. In reality, I recently celebrated my 30th year caring for the tiniest of miracles, and I wouldn't change it for the world. I have been truly blessed to have had an amazing career. I have witnessed the miracle of life, the tragedy of death, and the absolute resilience of these tiny humans.

As a new NICU nurse, I was thrust into the NICU world with a wonderful mentor who shaped me into who I am today. He was a wealth of information, pushed me to be my best, and was a trusted member of the NICU team. It was with him that I had my first experience of losing a precious patient. This sweet, premature girl was too tiny for this world, and I will never forget the grieving family, the sobs from her mother, and the tears that streamed down my face as I tried to understand how this could happen to such an innocent, tiny human. Unfortunately, I have witnessed many grieving families, but I will never forget sweet Samantha (name changed for privacy) and her will to live.

Thankfully, there has been more joy and happiness than sadness in my career. I have been privileged to witness thousands of babies leave through our front door and begin their journey with their families, who have become dear friends. I will never forget the first day that Eliza was able to be held by her sweet mom 2 months after her birthday to her going home day. I cherish hugs from my favorite 8-year-old (former 23-weeker), Lyndie, whom I will always cherish. And how can I forget the set of triplets, Abby, Parker, and Peyton, who were born at 22 weeks and 5 days and left a forever imprint on my heart? Peyton, the surviving triplet, is one of the most amazing humans I know.

I am truly blessed to have been a small part of the lives of all the NICU babies during my career. What an honor it is that their parents put their trust in me to care for the most important thing in their lives. I have touched so many tiny lives, but they have also touched me. And for that, I will be forever grateful.

Reflection Questions

1. Imagine yourself on the day of your retirement as a NICU nurse. How would you feel about the work you had done? Is there anything you would have wanted to do differently?
2. What do you think would be the biggest challenges of being a NICU nurse? How might you face these challenges?

PART III

Stories That Took a Piece of My Heart

How Could He Forget?

When I first started working in the NICU, I worked nights. I was the delivery room nurse for a 25-week little boy named Cooper (name changed for privacy). Cooper's time in the NICU did not go well. If anything bad was going to happen, it happened to Cooper. It seemed like he would take "one step forward and five steps back." Nothing went his way, and the worst part was that his parents lived a few hours away. They were visiting relatives when his mom went into labor and thus delivered at our hospital.

I became very attached to Cooper. In hindsight, I was probably too attached. I loved that little boy like he was my own. I even came in on nights I wasn't working to hold him because his mom could only come once a week. There is a lot we can do with traditional medicine, but a dose of love goes a long way in the healing process, and Cooper got a *lot* of love from me. I brought my Enya CD and would play it on repeat at his bedside. He loved it, but the nurses hated it. They said, "We cannot listen to one more Enya song!" One night, they hid the CD from me, but I still found it and played it. As a side note, through the years, I became known for playing Enya at the bedside. There are likely many babies and families out there who hear an Enya song and are instantly transported back to the NICU. I hope that is a good thing.

As Cooper got older (he was in our NICU for 6½ months), he started eating baby food. He was terrible about eating his vegetables. However, when I fed him, he always ate them. I also wore shoes that squeaked when I walked, and Cooper knew the squeak. He would turn his head to look toward me when he heard me coming. We had a special bond.

The time finally came for Cooper to go home. His parents were *so* excited. I still remember caring for him that night while he stayed in the "rooming out" room with them. He would cling to me and didn't want to go to his mom. When his mom would hold him, he would scream until she handed him to me. This was not a good situation. I reassured her that it was just because he was around me a lot and that he would come around. He was her son. That night, I gave his mom a brand-new Enya CD and told her that when Cooper was really upset, to play Enya. Enya seemed to make everything better for him. (Don't worry, I kept my Enya CD so that I could continue to play it for other babies and irritate the other nurses. Hehe.)

On my way home after discharging Cooper, I cried. I cried because I knew I was going to miss him. He was the first baby I had taken care of from delivery to discharge. I cared for him every night I worked (and even nights I wasn't working) for 6½ months. We aren't supposed to get attached, but that was impossible for me. I would randomly just start crying, wondering if Cooper missed me. I wanted to visit him at his house but didn't think it would be appropriate.

Then came the famous NICU reunion party. Every year, our NICU held a reunion for all the past NICU graduates to attend. I personally mailed out Cooper's invitation and was beyond excited to see the RSVP come back as "attending"! I was *so* excited about seeing Cooper. I had missed him so much, and it had been about 4 months since he was discharged home. I kept looking every time the door opened to see if it was Cooper, and finally, the time had arrived. I walked/ran to the door to see him, threw open my arms, and that's when he looked at me and then turned around to look at his mom and cried. I didn't know what to do. I stood there in shock. His mom tried handing him to me, but he screamed and flailed in my arms to return to his mom. I even talked to him in my "special" baby voice, which he had heard for 6½ months, but it didn't work. Cooper didn't remember me. How could this be?

The mom profusely apologized, to which I explained it wasn't her fault. This was how it was supposed to be, and I was so glad to see they had such a great connection. She told me that sometimes when he would be fussy in the car, she would put in the Enya CD, and he would instantly quiet and look around. I thought to myself, "He was looking for 'his Valerie.'" I finished up the conversation and then went to the bathroom and cried. I actually couldn't stop crying. Perhaps, it was all the infertility hormones I was on, but regardless, I was not in any shape to go back to the party. So, I snuck out the back and went home, crying the entire way.

Fast forward to 2006, when I was in the ICU as a patient. I received several get-well cards, but one of my favorites was from a little boy named Cooper. He had handwritten in the sweetest little boy's handwriting, "Get Well Valerie." I don't have contact with his mom—hence the need to change his name for privacy—but if I did, I would love to see him again. At the time I was writing this book, he would be 23 years old, which is crazy to think about. Wherever you are, Cooper, you will always hold a special place in my heart, as you were my first NICU love.

Reflection Questions

1. Valerie mentions an Enya CD that she liked to play for patients. Is there a song or an album you would want to use in similar situations?
2. Have you ever gotten attached to someone like Valerie got attached to Cooper? How did it make you feel when you were separated?

It Wasn't Supposed to Happen

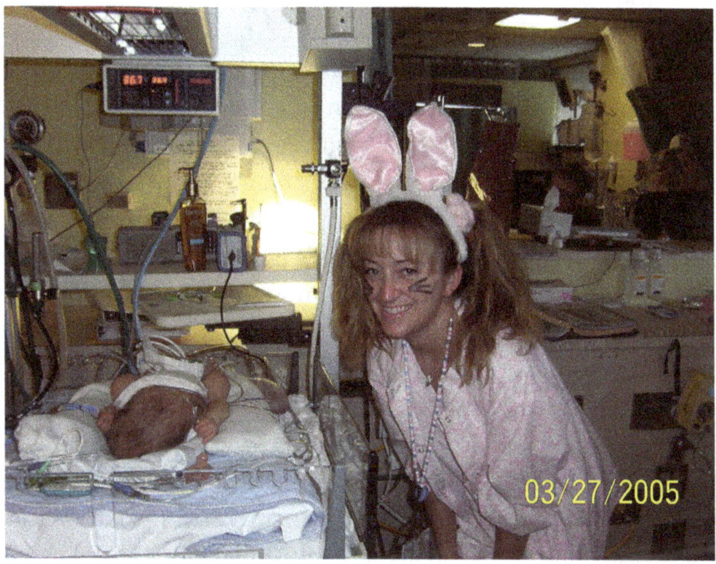

IMG 3.1

January 19, 2005, was a cold winter night, and our NICU was bursting at the seams. As the charge nurse, I had been begging for us to close, as we had no open beds available for admissions, very little remaining equipment, and staffing was really tight. We finally got the approval to close the NICU, which was a *huge* deal. When a NICU closes, that means they must divert all incoming admissions to surrounding hospitals that are open. This decision is never made lightly and is reassessed at least every 12 hours. The goal is never to close.

I remember feeling such a sigh of relief. Unfortunately, that relief was short-lived, as L&D called to let us know they were bringing a 30-week mom of twins, by helicopter, to our hospital. I fought with the L&D nurse, telling her how that wasn't allowed because we were closed. Apparently, though, the transfer was already in motion before our closing. The L&D nurse assured me they would stabilize her, and the twins wouldn't be born. Silly me for believing her.

We were nearing the end of the shift, and I was preparing assignments for the next shift when I got the call that they were taking the "twin mom" back to the OR to deliver the twins. I threw the biggest fit *ever*—like a toddler in the candy aisle—and yet there was absolutely nothing I could do about it. Even when scrubbing into the OR for the delivery, I thought, "This wasn't supposed to happen." But happen it did. Two perfect little 30-week baby boys were born that night, and by the grace of God, we found room for them—because, as a nurse, that's what you do. You figure it out. As we wheeled the twins to the NICU, I had no idea how much these boys and their family would impact my life. Forever.

Mason and Miles were chubby for 30-weekers, and initially, they did really well. One day, we were able to get them both out together. Mason was sleeping, and Miles was rooting around, and as if it was rehearsed, Mason reached his hand over, and Miles began sucking on his finger. It was a picture-perfect moment. I still have the actual picture we took of this precious moment. When I look at it, I think to myself, "*This* was how life was supposed to be for these boys," but unfortunately, that was not the reality.

Mason and Miles did so well, and after about 10 days, they transitioned from their isolettes to a crib together. Seeing twins reunited in a crib was such a priceless moment to have the opportunity to witness, and this time was no different. Except, shortly after moving them to the crib together, Miles began not looking "right." It is really hard to explain, but as an experienced NICU nurse, you could tell when something was just "off" with a baby, especially one you had cared for a lot. This is one time I wish I weren't right.

After several tests, we discovered that Miles had necrotizing enterocolitis (NEC). NEC is a serious gastrointestinal condition where bacteria causes inflammation of the gut lining, and when it progresses, it can actually cause the intestine to perforate, which means there is now a hole in the intestine. This hole allows bacteria and potentially the bowel contents to leak into the abdomen. This is never a good sign.

We were able to stabilize Miles, and although the NEC didn't progress to a perforation, it also didn't get any better. Our team of physicians and nurse practitioners, along with Miles's parents, decided to transport him to another hospital to have his patent ductus arteriosus (PDA) repaired. A PDA is a normal part of intrauterine circulation for a baby but should close shortly after birth. Because Miles still had a PDA, we were hoping that was the reason his NEC was not healing, and so repairing the PDA could, in fact, help the NEC. He was transported to another hospital, which was harder for me than I expected. I had become very close with the Penn family, especially with Miles. I took care of him almost every day I worked. So, giving up "control" to another hospital to care for our sweet Miles was hard. I remember crying on my way home that night. I also prayed for God to keep him safe at the other hospital and ultimately to heal him.

The surgery to repair his PDA went really well, and yet the NEC was not healing. At this point, Miles was in another hospital about 90 miles away, and Mason had progressed so well that he was ready to go home. In a perfect world, we would have just kept him in the NICU until his family returned, but insurance simply doesn't allow it. As we prepared Mason to go home with his parents, we luckily worked it out with the insurance company for Miles to return to his "home" NICU. The terrible thing about this is that once a baby is discharged, they are not allowed back into the NICU. This means their parents would have to split up their visiting time: one in the waiting room with Mason and one in the NICU with Miles. This is not an ideal situation, ever.

I had hoped that Miles would improve once back "home" in our NICU, especially with his repaired PDA, but he did not. He, unfortunately, got worse. His intestines began to perforate in multiple places, and we had to take him to the OR more than once to repair them. One of the times we were in the OR, I would call Miles's dad, Tyler, to give him an update. Each time I called, I gave Tyler the update that things were going pretty well, but then things took a turn. I remember dreading calling him. I had dialed the phone and hung up more than once before I finally had the courage to give him the bad news that the surgeon ultimately couldn't repair the damage. I finally got up the courage, and when Tyler answered, he knew something was wrong by my voice, even though I tried to keep my voice the same as it always was. I thought to myself that I could "fake it" more over the phone, but I guess I was wrong. We stabilized him in the OR and brought him back to the NICU. I cried in the OR. I cried as we transported him back to the NICU. I had to "get it together" before we got back and saw his parents, which was basically impossible. Miles was critical but stable.

One day I had picked him up to change his linens in the warmer, and his orogastric (OG) tube leaked green gastric contents all down my back. Usually, I would be *super* grossed out by this. Heck, I'd probably even gag and maybe even throw up. Ironically, as a nurse, I could do urine, feces, and vomit, but not mucous stuff that came from the mouth, like spit—and especially not green spit. I remember someone saying that you could tell the difference between a nurse and a respiratory therapist by hypothetically putting them both in a pool of poop up to their waist, then dumping a bucket of mucous over their heads. The respiratory therapist would stand up and take it, and the nurses would dunk themselves down in the poo. Anyway, it was really at this point that I realized how much I loved sweet baby Miles—because I didn't even care. I remember his parents commenting on it: how I had "grown up" as a nurse not to be grossed out by it. I didn't say anything at the time, but if it were any other baby, I would have been grossed out by it, but because I was so attached to Miles, there was nothing he could do to gross me out.

I can still remember how when Miles was critically ill, I put him in his bouncy seat in the warmer. This was really unheard of; however, I wanted him to experience something that babies get to do: bounce in a bouncy seat. It brought a sense of normalcy to this unfathomable situation. I would like to think that Miles loved it. Even though it was against the rules, I also "snuck" Mason in to see his brother. Little did I know it would be the last time.

Toward the end, we struggled to keep Miles in a stable condition. It was so hard. I remember his mom, Kellie, singing "Jesus Loves Me" at his bedside. I am not sure who can witness this and not break down. I had worked to perfect my ability to cry and not let anyone know. Sometimes, I would go out and break down in the supply closet, as if somehow the medical supplies could console my brokenness. In reality, I wasn't fooling anyone. With my red face and puffy eyes, I would continue caring for Miles. I even picked up extra shifts so that I would be the one caring for him, as if I had some magical power that was keeping him alive. I have never worked so many back-to-back shifts in my life. On my last shift with Miles, I worked 18 hours, planning to come back the next day and do it all over again. But God had a different plan. On April 22, 2005, Miles went to his final home with Jesus. I had only been home for a few hours when I got the call that he died. I knew when the phone rang in the early hours of the morning that it was not good. I remember thinking that I wouldn't answer the phone, as if not answering it would keep it from being a reality. I also remember feeling so guilty. I even carry a bit of that guilt with me to this day. I thought he wouldn't have died if I had been there with him. But in reality, I wonder if he waited until I was gone—if God somehow knew I wasn't strong enough to be there. To this day, I will never know.

I quickly got dressed and came back to the NICU to help with Miles's final care and to be with his family. I cried and cried and cried. I really shouldn't have been driving. To this day, I think God actually drove me to work that day. I helped with his final bath. I helped with his final footprints, and I handed him to his parents for the last time. Even as I write out this story, I am crying. I loved sweet Miles and his family so much. My heart broke for them. They were good people, and bad stuff isn't supposed to happen to good people, but that's not how life works. This is at the top of my list of things to talk to God about when I get to Heaven.

The day after Miles died, I returned to work as the charge nurse. I can still remember it to this day; the sun was shining down on

Miles's empty bed—directly on his bed. It was like he was sending me a message from Heaven that he was okay. He was finally healed. I couldn't stop crying, and yet I was expected to go about my day like it was any other day. I remember keeping Miles's bed open. I refused to admit another baby into "his" bed. I even got "talked to" because I was so adamant about it. Then one night, they admitted another baby into Miles's bed, as it was our last available bed. When I came to work the next day, I was furious. It was irrational, I know, to think that we could always keep that bed open. However, it hit me so hard to see another baby in his bed. These are things that you don't really think about—until they happen.

We ended up having counselors from our hospital Employee Assistance Program come to talk with the nurses. Although I was one of Miles's primary nurses, others took care of him, and anybody that knew the Penn family instantly loved them. Miles's death rocked our NICU to its core. There were times in my career as a NICU nurse when my own mental health or the mental health of my colleagues was not prioritized, but it was definitely prioritized after the death of Miles—mostly because we were struggling to carry on with our regular responsibilities. Talking with the counselors, and each other, helped us cope. We also went together and bought little fish aquariums that played lullaby music (one of Miles's favorite things) and donated them to the NICU for other babies to enjoy and as a permanent reminder of Miles's precious time on this Earth.

In all seriousness, to this day, it is impossible to put into words how much the life of sweet baby Miles changed my life. I circle back to the title of this story, "This Wasn't Supposed to Happen," but now I realize it was all part of a bigger plan. Because of Miles and his parents, I gave my life to Jesus. My life here on Earth, and eternally, was forever changed because of Miles. His 3 short months on this Earth planted the seed that has changed the lives of many, including myself, and for that, I will be forever grateful.

To hear more about the story of Kellie and Tyler Penn and their sweet babies, check out the podcast *The Unfolding*. The episode is titled "Kellie Penn."

Reflection Questions

1. What feelings did this story bring up?
2. There is more literature out now regarding NEC prevention. What are some of the advances in science, specifically regarding NEC, that have occurred since 2005?
3. As the nurse, how would you have managed Mason's inability to come to the NICU? Would you have done things differently than Valerie? If so, how?
4. If you had the chance, would you have put Miles in the bouncy seat? Why, or why not?

Our Tiniest Little Fighter

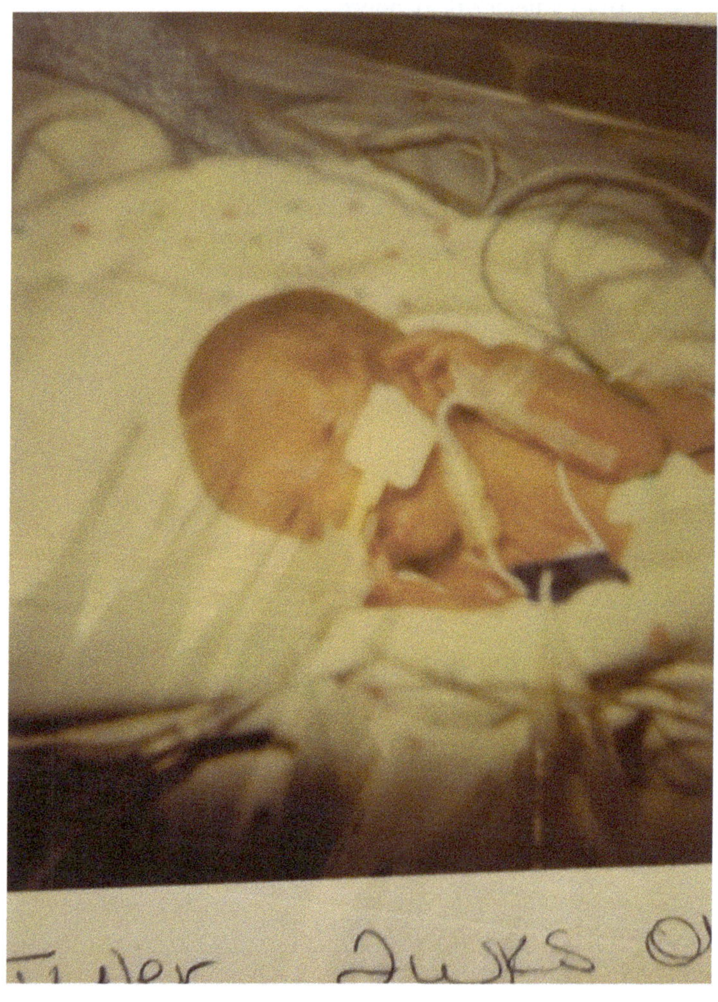

IMG 3.2

Tyler was born on August 16, 2002. He was 23 and 5/7 weeks gestation when he was born and weighed a lofty 1 pound, 6 ounces. While I was not at his delivery, I was his primary nurse during his time in our NICU. I remember Tyler was the tiniest little fighter. Typically, babies born less than 24 weeks gestation really struggle to survive and often only live a few days. Tyler was different, though.

I routinely took care of the tiny babies, and so caring for Tyler was a typical assignment for me. I took care of him and his family each day I worked. I was initially surprised at how well Tyler was doing. We all were, as he seemed to really be defying the odds. As NICU nurses, we care for each baby we are assigned to, but I especially cared for Tyler, and it was such a privilege to watch him fight so hard.

I am still in contact with Tyler's mom. When I reached out to her to get permission to use Tyler's name in this story, she reminded me about one of the times when she came to visit. She had been to visit a lot, and I knew she wasn't taking care of herself; specifically, I knew she wasn't really eating. So, I asked her to get something to eat and reassured her that I would take the very best care of her son until she returned.

As the days progressed, Tyler's condition started to get more critical. He fought harder. We fought harder. But unfortunately, it wasn't enough. On September 11, 2002, Tyler passed away in his mother's arms. I stayed 6 hours after my shift was over caring for Tyler and ultimately for them as they grieved the loss of their son. I couldn't have imagined being anywhere else.

I remembered feeling guilty, like I had failed Tyler as a nurse. Logic doesn't always come into play when your heart is broken. This was early on in my career, and I really had no framework for how to deal with my grief. Caring for babies so much and then watching them die was incomprehensible. Sometimes, I'd cry in the supply closet. Sometimes, I'd even cry at the bedside, my tears streaming down onto the bed as I hoped they might have some special power to save the baby I was caring for.

A few weeks later, Tyler's parents returned to the NICU and asked to see me. I came to the front desk, and they had a small, wrapped gift for me. I had no idea what to say. This had never happened. I was not sure why they were giving me a gift when I felt as if I failed them as Tyler's nurse. I opened the gift to find a porcelain nurse. The nurse was on top of a wind-up music box that played the sweetest tune. It also had an inscription that read, "As I care for my patients today, bless me with kindness in all I do and say." As they thanked me again for going above and beyond as Tyler's nurse, I told them, "It's my job." But you know what, it wasn't "just" a job for me. It never was. I did go above and beyond because I loved those babies, every one of them I cared for, but especially Tyler.

I still have that porcelain nurse. She sits on my desk to remind me that nursing has never been and will never be "just my job." Even as I have transitioned my career into teaching, I still give it my all. It's who I am. And Tyler and his family helped me to realize that what I did was special, and that is something I will be forever grateful for.

Reflection Questions

1. Have you ever felt like a "failure" even when there was no logical reason for you to? If so, why do you think you felt that way?
2. How are you prepared to handle instances where no matter how hard you try, you can't save a patient? What coping mechanisms and self-care rituals do you utilize during times of stress and despair?

One Last Picture

We got the call in the NICU that a 34-week mom had been in a terrible car accident and had a life-threatening injury. They kept her alive until she arrived at the hospital, but barely. I was the delivery nurse at the emergency C-section. The baby had heart tones before the delivery, but they quickly dropped. We had our entire resuscitation team at the delivery, which we unfortunately needed.

The initial steps of neonatal resuscitation weren't enough, and we ultimately had to begin chest compressions and provide assisted ventilation. It felt like it was all going in slow motion, despite being ridiculously fast-paced and hectic. At this point, trauma surgeons took over the surgery. We were able to stabilize the baby and take her to the NICU. However, as we left the operating room, I heard the surgeons ask for the defibrillator and scream, "CLEAR!" It's like something you see in the movies, but this was, unfortunately, real life.

We stabilized the baby in the NICU and ultimately got her off the ventilator. Despite her rocky start, she was doing really well. Unfortunately, her mom was not. We got the news that they would not be able to save the mom. She was an organ donor, so they were awaiting the arrival of UNOS (United Network for Organ Sharing). I knew the mom was in the adult ICU at our hospital and called up to talk to her nurse. I asked if I could bring the baby to the ICU to get pictures with the mom before she passed. The nurse agreed, and so I packed up the baby in the transport isolette and went to the adult ICU. With the help of the mom's nurse, the baby's father, and myself, we took pictures of this precious baby with her mom. I remember crying on the way to the ICU. I just couldn't comprehend how painful this was for the family and how this little girl would feel growing up having never been able to know her mommy. These pictures were important, as they would be the only memento this little girl would have with her and her mom together.

The mom had several injuries, and there was still dried blood on her face and hair, as well as her arms and hands. I took a washcloth and gently cleaned away the blood. I wasn't able to get all of the blood off, especially in her hair. I vividly remember covering up some of her bloodied hair with one of the baby blankets, as I didn't want the little girl to see it when she looked back at the pictures of her with her mom. I could barely look at it, and she wasn't my mom. Through tears in our eyes, we took pictures of this precious baby girl with her mom, as well as some with the mom and dad. I can't begin to fathom how heartbreaking this experience was for this family.

As a nurse, it is hard for me to separate my personal feelings from my feelings as a nurse. I would often put myself in the place of the person who was going through something horrific, and at times it was more than I could bear. Merriam-Webster defines empathy as "the action of understanding, being aware of, being sensitive to, and vicariously experiencing the feelings, thoughts, and experiences of another."[1] Well, God gave me an extra dose of empathy, which made seeing things like this especially hard. I could have avoided it by not suggesting the pictures, but that wouldn't have been right. This little baby girl, who would now be in her 20s, has these pictures as a keepsake of the first and last time she was with her mom. I don't remember her name, but to whoever you are, know it was a privilege to share these precious moments with you and your family. May you look back at these pictures and know how much your mommy loved you.

---

1 *Merriam-Webster*, s.v. "Empathy (n.)," accessed July 2, 2023, https://www.merriam-webster.com/dictionary/empathy.

Reflection Questions

1. What is one key takeaway you have after reading this story?
2. Valerie mentions the importance of mementos for the baby to have to remember their mother. Besides pictures, is there anything you can think of that could act as a special memento?
3. The weight of this story is indescribable. How might you have personally coped if you were in Valerie's shoes?

There's No Heartbeat

I answered the phone like I always did: "NICU, this is Valerie." The nurse from L&D said, "We need you now! The baby's got no heartbeat!" I could hear screaming in the background. I'm not sure whether I hung up the phone before I yelled for our nurse practitioner to come with me to the room in L&D. One of the other nurses called our NICU respiratory therapist (RT) and told them to meet us in L&D *stat*.

We ran as fast as we could to the room we were called to—sprinted actually. They had the door open and were waiting for us. Luckily, our NICU was on the same floor as L&D, so we didn't have far to go. It is interesting to watch movies where healthcare workers are running to the scene; they arrive and aren't even out of breath. Let me tell you, this was not the case. You see, getting the call that there's no heartbeat gets your heartbeat going pretty fast; then we sprinted to the room, and by the time we arrived, we were completely out of breath—nothing like the movies.

Sometimes when we are called like this, we get to the room and the baby is fine. In cases like that, the staff had difficulty initially finding a heartbeat, and the baby ultimately turned around. Unfortunately, this time they were right. When we ran in, the obstetrician was at the baby's warmer, doing chest compressions with tears running down her face. The RT was right behind us, and we immediately got to work.

The room we were in was very small. I could have reached out and touched the mom; that's how close the warmer was to the parents. The lack of space made it difficult to perform the resuscitation, but we made do with what we had. I ended up squeezing in on the side of the warmer, between the warmer and the wall. To complicate matters, the parents had to witness the entire resuscitation. Right after delivery is when the mom and dad get to snuggle with their newborn, and the complete opposite was happening to this sweet family as they watched us resuscitate their precious daughter. I remember them begging us to save her. I remember the obstetrician holding the mom's hand as she cried herself, telling her we were doing everything we could.

We started with the initial steps of resuscitation and went all the way down the NRP algorithm. Still no heartbeat. The 1-minute Apgar was zero. Anesthesiologist Virginia Apgar developed the evaluation, and it stands for appearance, pulse, grimace, activity, and respiration. Babies are given a score from zero to two for each category, with the highest score being ten and the lowest zero. APGAR scores don't dictate our care; the baby's response to our resuscitation efforts dictates the care. It is, however, something we document in every delivery.

It is very normal for the 1-minute APGAR to be between seven and ten and the same at 5 minutes. Not only was this baby's 1-minute Apgar zero, but the 5-minute APGAR was also zero. Our resuscitation efforts continued: chest compressions, intubation and ventilation—still nothing. The baby's color was pale grey and, despite our interventions, never changed.

We always do everything we can, but sometimes it isn't enough. We quickly got an umbilical line placed. We continued with round after round of epinephrine. Still no response. The 10-minute APGAR was zero. We began doing boluses of normal saline. You see, the baby's color was a pale grey, which would normally indicate blood loss; however, the mom had not hemorrhaged during the delivery. The baby had great heart tones during and up to the delivery. Something wasn't right.

We called our neonatologist because, back then, neonatologists weren't in-house, so not only were we on the phone with him during the beginning part of the resuscitation but he also then had to drive across town while talking to us on his flip cell phone. I still remember pulling the phone cord in the delivery room as far as it would go to be closer to the bed. This also meant that the cord went across the mom, as the phone was on the wall on the other side of the delivery bed. The L&D nurse was the one relaying to us what the neonatologist was saying, which, again, was right over the mom. It was incomprehensible.

We had been resuscitating for 20 minutes and still had no heartbeat. Normally, at 20 minutes, we would stop. However, back then, neonatal nurse practitioners could not call the time of death. It had to be done by a physician. We continued resuscitation until our neonatologist arrived, and at 22 minutes, we got a faint heartbeat with an APGAR score of two. It was something, and so we continued. We noticed the most improvement after giving the saline boluses, so we continued giving them. I just remember drawing up syringe after syringe and administering them. I would have done it for days if that is what it would have taken.

We got the heart rate up enough to transport the baby girl to the NICU. We had called ahead and ordered STAT blood, which was waiting when we arrived. I hung the blood transfusion. Then I hung another blood transfusion. I don't know how many I did, but finally, the baby's color slowly changed from pale grey to pale pink. Pink always has been and will always be my favorite color.

The baby's condition became more stable as the days went on. She had a tracheotomy to help her breathe and a feeding tube placed for feedings. And eventually, she went home. However, this was not the baby girl the parents had planned on taking home. She would need around-the-clock care, likely for the rest of her life. My heart broke for this sweet family.

Looking back, there was so much going on in such a short amount of time. As a nurse, I would try to disassociate myself from the emotions of it all to focus on my job. That might work for some nurses, but it never worked for me. You see, you can't ignore the emotions. If you don't deal with them at the time, they will come up later, like during the drive home, at 2:00 a.m. while lying in bed, or in the middle of a movie. Either way, they will come up.

I like to use the analogy of emotions flowing in the body like a continuous body of water, almost like a river. Each time an emotion comes up that we don't deal with, we put a hypothetical rock in our hypothetical river of emotions. One or two rocks are not a big deal, but they add up quickly, and eventually, the emotions will burst through. The funny thing is that the incident that caused the "burst" likely had nothing to do with the real reason; it was just the final rock in an otherwise large pile of rocks—sitting there, never dealt with.

When I started as a nurse, I didn't fully realize the repercussions of pushing back my emotions. I am not saying I should have dealt with them in the delivery room, but I certainly should have allowed space for them afterward when the situation was over and I was no longer responsible for the life I was supposed to save. I look back at situations like this one and wonder how I did it, day after day, week after week, year after year. I also wonder about the babies and their families I cared for, especially this one.

Reflection Questions

1. What are your thoughts surrounding the ethics of this story?
2. How do you deal with your emotions when they come up? Have you ever had them "burst"?

Gone Too Soon

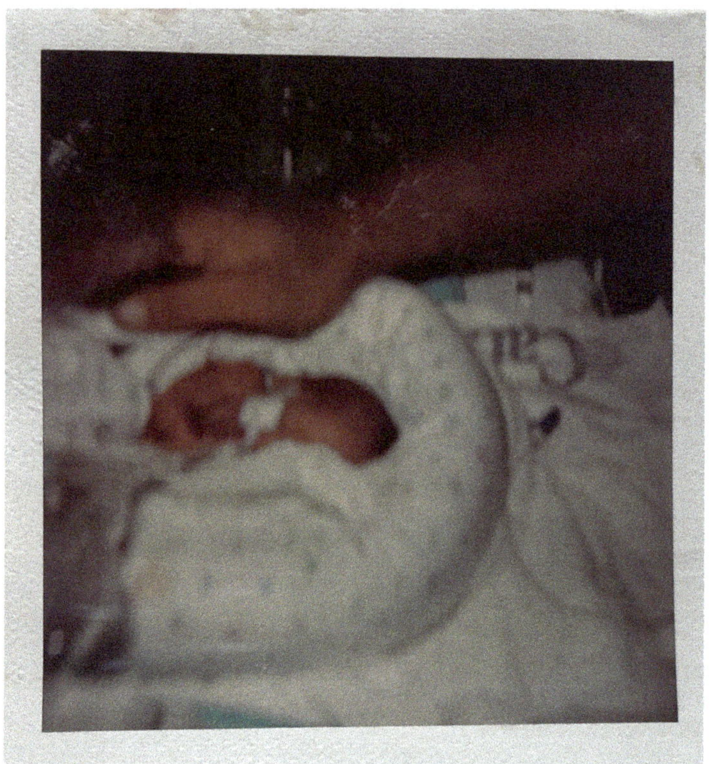

IMG 3.3

On September 19, 2002, my cousin Megan Harley was born at the hospital where I worked. My aunt had placental previa and had to be on bed rest for about a month. In the last few weeks, she was admitted to the hospital, as she had quite a bit of bleeding. Luckily, she was at the hospital when her placenta ultimately detached from her uterus (placental abruption), thus causing the need for an emergency C-section. Megan was born just shy of 24 weeks and weighed 623 grams (1 pound, 4 ounces).

I remembered getting the call that my aunt was being taken back for an emergency C-section, and I knew it was too soon. There are times when, as a nurse, you wish you didn't have the knowledge you have, especially when the information isn't good and ultimately affects you and/or your family. This was one of those times.

For obvious reasons, I was not Megan's nurse. I remember being at the hospital, though, and trying to answer my family's questions. I remembered trying to soften the news that Megan was not doing well. This was something I had done several times as a NICU nurse, but there was something about it being my own family that made it remarkably harder. I remember making the cutest little name card for Megan—in pink, of course. I am also certain I would have put a bow in her hair, even if she didn't have any, because every little girl deserves a bow.

Because Megan was unstable, they decided to bring my aunt into the NICU in the hospital bed. I always hated when we had to bring moms to visit when they were in the hospital bed because it was basically impossible for them to see the baby, especially if we couldn't move the baby due to all the wires and tubes. It was better than nothing, but certainly not ideal.

This was the first time my family had been to the NICU. They knew where I worked but didn't *really* know what it was like, until now. I remember the oddness of looking up and seeing my uncle, dad, and grandma in the NICU. In my mind, I had done a good job of separating my job from my family, so having Megan in the NICU I worked at was especially hard to wrap my mind around.

As Megan's condition worsened, we discovered she had a severe intraventricular hemorrhage (bleeding into her brain). This type of news is incomprehensible for the baby's family, but now I was not "just" the nurse; I was also a part of the family. My heart broke for my aunt and uncle. In times like this, there really are no words to make it better. Little did I know that in just a few years, I would know this same feeling, except this time with my own daughter and son.

After speaking with our neonatologist, my aunt and uncle made the unfathomable decision to remove Megan from life support. This is a decision no parent should ever have to make, and it never got easier to watch, no matter how many times I witnessed it over the years. They were able to hold her and say their final goodbyes as she breathed her last breath in their arms. We had a private room that families could use, and I remember being in that room with my family. It was almost an out-of-body experience. We each had the opportunity to hold Megan for the first and last time. It was precious yet utterly devastating, especially for my aunt and uncle.

It is almost impossible to find the "bright side" in situations like these, but because of our faith, we know we will see Megan again. I often think about Megan in Heaven, playing with other babies called Home too soon, including Joey and Callie. One day, we will be with them all again, and oh, what a glorious day that will be.

Reflection Questions

1. What are three emotions you can name after reading this story?
2. Do you think having medical knowledge makes situations like these easier or more difficult? Explain your answer.

As Many Times as It Takes

I was working the night shift, and at the beginning of my shift, I was assigned to a baby boy who was actively dying. Within the first hour, the baby, unfortunately, passed away. Most times, when we are assigned babies at the beginning of the shift, we are assigned more than one, but in this circumstance, I was fortunate to only have this little boy and his family.

The mom was still in the postpartum unit in a private room, which thankfully provided the space they needed as they grieved a loss that no parent should ever have to grieve. Together, in their room, we did his handprints and footprints, gave him his last bath, dressed him in the sweetest little outfit, swaddled him up, took pictures, and allowed them to say their final goodbyes. I left the room and told them to call me when they were ready for me to take their son. I wanted to ensure they had as much time as they needed.

About an hour later, they called me and said they were done. With tears in their eyes and mine, I took the baby back to the NICU. What came next was the least favorite part of my job. I had to take the baby to the morgue. I cannot begin to describe how dreadful this process was, and it never got easier.

I kept the baby swaddled, put him in a crib, covered the crib with a blanket, and pushed the crib to the elevator and ultimately to the basement where the morgue was. I didn't like putting the babies in the crib and covering it, but that was really the only option. I couldn't carry them, for fear that someone in the elevator would ask to see the baby. This was the same reason we covered the cribs with a blanket: so everyone just thought we were transporting a clean crib.

Even as I write this, I can still see the morgue in extreme detail. I see all the stainless steel and can even smell the smells. And that isn't the worst part. The worst part was having to leave a precious baby on that metal table all alone. It went against everything I was ever taught, and every time I had to do it, it ripped out a tiny piece of my heart. Those pieces can never be replaced. So, when people say to me, "Working in the NICU must have been so much fun. You got to play with babies all day," I would typically lose it. If one considered this "playing with babies," their idea of fun differed greatly from mine. Of course, I know people don't really think taking a baby to the morgue is fun; they simply don't know what the job fully entails—until now.

Back to this specific time, I lingered in the morgue, holding the baby and crying, telling myself that I had to leave him. It was my job. And I hated it with every fiber of my being. You never leave babies on a table alone, especially on a cold table. They shouldn't be left with strangers either, but that is what you have to do. It's almost impossible to explain, but there is such a strange feeling in the morgue—a palpable emptiness. I wonder if it is because there are bodies in the morgue, but their human souls have gone to Heaven. You have to be in the room to experience it, and it is my hope for you that this never happens.

I pulled it together as much as possible, laid him down, and then pushed the empty crib back to NICU. I went back to the parents' room and let them know to call me if there was anything I could do. Usually, I don't get a call, but this night, I did. Some of their family had come from out of town and wanted to see the baby, so I took the crib back to the morgue and got the baby. I carried with me a bottle of Johnson & Johnson baby shampoo, smeared a bit of it on the blanket to cover up the smell of the morgue, placed the baby under the infant warmer bed for a few minutes, then took the baby back to the room. Over the course of the night, this happened a total of six different times.

After that night, when I was in a similar situation, I would tell the parents something like this, "You call me as much as you need. Once, I went back to get a baby six times for a family, and I would have done it 100 times if it had helped them. There's not a number that is too much. It's whatever you need. Period." With that said, people grieve differently, and as a nurse and a human, it is our job not to judge the process. We are to be there and provide space for them to process their own grief, however that may look. I specifically remember telling them I would do it as many times as it took for them to feel complete. Of course, they would never feel totally complete, as part of them was gone—forever.

In closing, there is something about being discharged from the hospital as a postpartum mom and not having your baby to hold. Every mom should have the opportunity to be wheeled to their car, holding their precious child in their arms. In cases where the baby passed away, we would give the mom a pink or blue teddy bear. While this did not console their grief, it gave them something to hold onto as they left the hospital, leaving behind their precious child and a piece of their heart. This is why, after Joey and Callie died, we donated pink and blue bears to the NICU and continued to do so for years afterward. If you are reading this and you have one of those bears, it is my hope and prayer that it helped to provide some sort of peace during such a tragic time in your life. And if your baby died and you didn't receive a bear, I am so sorry. Please know that although you couldn't carry your baby home, they will live on forever inside your heart, bear or no bear.

Reflection Questions

1. How might you have responded when asked to go get the baby back from the morgue?
2. What feelings came up for you when you read about how Valerie had to leave the baby in the morgue?
3. Valerie mentions that many people mistakenly believe working in the NICU means getting to "play with babies all day." What are some aspects of the job you think people don't think about? Are there any that surprised you or that you would be nervous about performing?

Not Your Routine C-Section

I was the delivery nurse and attended the routine morning C-section delivery. This was back when we attended routine C-section deliveries with the pediatrician who was on-call. As they were preparing the mom, the nurse came and told us that they hadn't heard heart tones in a while, but it was due to her larger size. They had previously been checking heart tones via a vaginal ultrasound, but the last one recorded was a month ago. Due to her size, the mom also had difficulty feeling the baby move.

I quickly looked over at our code box and undid the lock on it so it would be ready. I figured if I was prepared, we wouldn't need it. Unfortunately, I was wrong. The delivery took longer than expected, and when the baby was finally born, there was only silence, which is never what you want to hear in the delivery room.

We quickly got the baby to the warmer and began the initial steps for resuscitation; however, it was clear that something wasn't right. As I dried the baby, his skin was sluffing off. In addition to this, the smell was like nothing I had ever experienced. None of this was normal.

The pediatrician and I began chest compressions while the L&D nurse called the NICU for backup. Our neonatologist came along with our neonatal nurse practitioner and respiratory therapist. We did everything we could but were never able to get a heartbeat. It was absolutely gut-wrenching.

I can still hear the mom sobbing as the OB team kept her informed. She was also set to have a tubal ligation, which they were waiting for to see if we could save her little boy. After our neonatologist called the time of death, the mom decided not to do the tubal. We wrapped up her little boy and brought him to her so she could hold him. There was nothing routine about this delivery. In hindsight, the providers felt like the baby might have been gone for quite some time. Because she couldn't feel the baby move and they weren't routinely checking heart tones, they weren't sure exactly how long.

I remember leaving the OR that morning with such a heavy feeling. I also struggled to get the smell out of my nose. One of the experienced nurses told me about a trick to go get Vicks from the pharmacy and put some in my nose, which I did, and it helped. But the Vicks didn't help the images from continuing to flash through my mind or the sounds of the mom sobbing. And this was all before 8:00 a.m.. I still had an assignment I had to go back to, babies that needed cared for. That was one of the hardest parts of being a NICU nurse. You have to go from seeing something so incomprehensibly sad to changing a healthy baby's diaper and talking to their mom about their upcoming circumcision—from a tragically sad assignment to an overwhelmingly happy one, all within just minutes.

I learned over the years to allow space to process the sad encounters, even if just for 5 minutes. It wasn't fair to bring that unprocessed grief to my next patient and their family. Sometimes, I processed it in an empty room; sometimes, the supply closet. Actually, most of the time was the supply closet. The gauze packages and diapers didn't judge my ugly cry, and there was always a full box of Kleenex ready to take it on.

Reflection Questions

1. Imagine being in a similar situation and then being assigned another patient load. What would you do to clear your head and prepare for the next patient?
2. Is there anything that could have been done differently in this scenario? If so, what?

PART IV

The Lighter Side of the NICU

Don't Eat the Cookies

I used to have a personal "policy" that I never, ever ate what people brought into the NICU—unless it was in a sealed package. I just didn't trust people: What did they put in it? Was their kitchen clean? To me, it just wasn't worth eating it; plus, it wasn't like I was turning down something super healthy. I will never forget this one mom who kept bringing in homemade chocolate-chip cookies. She was an interesting character, and if my "rule" applied to anyone, it definitely applied to her. However, the nurses just kept raving about her chocolate-chip cookies, saying how good they were and trying to get me to eat one. It didn't matter how good they were; I would never eat one. One day, we were all sitting around the NICU feeding babies and one of the nurses asked this mom what her recipe was because her cookies were *so* good. The mom very proudly replied that her cookies were always better right after having a baby because she used breastmilk instead of regular milk as the "secret" ingredient. As she told the story, I watched the other nurses' faces—those who couldn't stop raving about the cookies. The look on their faces was priceless. I could also see a few of them subtly gag. How are the chocolate-chip cookies now, ladies? No, thank you. I'm still not interested, and I guarantee you they thought twice after that incident.

Reflection Questions

1. If you were one of the nurses sitting around the bedside and heard the mom say she used her own breastmilk in the cookies you ate, how would that have made you feel? How might you have responded?
2. Do you think you will eat homemade treats brought to the hospital during your career?

We've Got a Situation

In the NICU, we had a "rooming out" room that we used before babies were discharged home. Parents would come and stay the night with their babies before taking them home. This way, they could have a "dry run" with the NICU staff readily accessible. I was assigned the baby in the rooming out room and went out to check on the baby and parents. When I walked in, the mom was dying laughing and the dad was standing there in his boxers. Apparently, he went to the bathroom, and the toilet tipped over while he was sitting on it, so there was water and other "things" on the floor, and the dad was soaking wet. All I kept thinking was that I just came in to check on the baby. I had no idea what to do about this toilet situation except laugh. I laughed so hard that night, and the parents laughed too. I called maintenance, and they came to save the day—or, rather, the night. Apparently, the toilet was not bolted to the floor, and it was just a matter of time before it tipped over. I bet you that every time that dad sits on a toilet, he thinks twice and braces himself for the unknown.

Reflection Questions

1. What would your response have been walking into a similar situation?
2. When Valerie responded to this situation with laughter, how did that make you feel?

Never, Ever, Shake a Baby

While I was being precepted in the newborn nursery, we had one of the busiest nights ever. We had 14 babies in the nursery that night—most of which were screaming – but the moms didn't want them in the room because they wanted to sleep—and clearly, their baby wasn't sleeping. One baby, in particular, had a very high pitch shrill-like cry, and he was relentless. It didn't matter what we did, we couldn't soothe him. I thought to myself that these parents were going to lose their minds if he did this at home. Just then, my preceptor went over and picked up the baby—looked him right in the eyes, and said slowly and methodically, "Never, ever, shake a baby." Then she put the baby down slowly, looked over at me, and said, "I am going to go take a break." I remember this just like it was yesterday, and I replied with, "Okay, you do that, and when you get back, I am going."

Reflection Questions

1. Reflect on a situation you have been in which was overwhelming, like the scenario above.
2. What are your honest thoughts when you read about a caregiver saying, "Never, ever, shake a baby"?
3. Once home, what are strategies the parents could utilize to ensure they are safe around their baby?

Ma'am, Please Put on a Shirt

One of our NICU moms was extra "free" with her clothes; specifically, she would breastfeed and/or pump and then walk across the entire NICU—with no shirt or bra on—to wash her pumping supplies or sometimes to talk to another family. We had many complaints about her "free spirit" and told her repeatedly to put on a shirt before leaving the bedside. Ironically, she never saw the issue with it. It was the oddest thing to be walking through the NICU and have a mom approach you without a shirt or bra on. Not everyone minded, but still, we had to tell her it was not okay. I will never forget the day that a newly admitted baby's grandparents were visiting, and she walked right past them without a shirt or bra on. I am fairly certain their eyes had never been so big. To this day I can think back to their faces and laugh.

Reflection Questions

1. How would you have responded when seeing this mother walk through the NICU with no shirt or bra on?
2. Have you ever encountered an awkward situation like this? If so, what was it, and how did you respond?

Eyes, Thighs, and Triple Dye

When I worked in the NICU, after each baby was born, they were given "eyes, thighs, and triple dye" as a part of their routine care. The "eyes" part was erythromycin to prevent infection in the eyes. "Thighs" was vitamin K, as babies aren't born with a high level of vitamin K and need it to help with blood clotting. "Triple dye" was used to prevent infection and placed directly on the baby's umbilical cord. The triple dye came in an ampule that you squeezed, which then released the dark purple solution out of the top so that you could place it directly on the umbilical cord. One night, I popped the ampule, and the entire ampule came open (which had never happened and never happened again). All the solution in the ampule (like a dark purple dye) spilled out over the baby's abdomen. The more I tried to clean it up, the worse it got. Before I had a chance to talk to the parents about the "situation," they reported me to the unit manager for abusing their baby, as they thought I had bruised his entire abdomen. Clearly, this was not something I would do, but I understand how they could come to that assumption, as the belly looked severely bruised. The manager talked with the parents, explaining the situation, and ultimately, we all laughed together about it once it was over. From then on, I was extra careful with the triple dye ampules, and if it got on the belly at all, I warned the parents ahead of time.

Reflection Questions

1. Imagine yourself in these parents' shoes. How might you have responded?
2. Now imagine yourself in Valerie's shoes and reflect on how you would have responded.

Who Did It This Time?

We had a removable face on our baby CPR mannequin. Somebody had the brilliant idea to start pranking other nurses by placing just the face mask in random places: diaper drawers, medicine cabinets—just random places. You never knew where it would pop up next—that is, until the last time. Somebody took the mask and placed it on top of a stuffed monkey and wrapped it like a baby, then called another nurse over, saying that there was just something that didn't look "right" about the baby and that they wanted a second opinion. The nurse who was called over to the "baby" looked into the crib and screamed so loudly because, let's face it: The mask was *so* creepy. Luckily, this happened in the middle of the night, so no parents were around. Either way, though, we made the collective decision that the joke needed to end, but that night, we laughed until we cried. I often wonder if anyone since then has done the same thing. Probably not. We were a "special" group of night nurses.

Reflection Questions

1. What are some work shenanigans you've been a part of?
2. Do you think that pranks at work are a good idea or a bad idea? Why?
3. How would you have reacted if you were the nurse that found the stuffed monkey "baby"?

Middle of the Night Microwaving

At the NICU, we sanitized the bottles in a steam bag in the microwave. The microwave lived on a counter in the middle of the NICU, not near any babies—thank goodness. To sterilize the bottles, you had to microwave them on high for 4 minutes. One night, one of the nurses was exceptionally tired and set the microwave for 40 minutes instead of 4, and the microwave ended up exploding the door open, making a HUGE banging sound. Several of us screamed, thinking it was a bomb, and it kind of was: a bottle bomb inside the microwave. The microwave was ruined after that, as the door came completely off. The bottles and nipples were also ruined as they completely melted. Afterward, we had a note on the microwave with a reminder for how many minutes to set it for when sanitizing bottles and their nipples. The moral of the story is that zeros matter when setting the "cooking time" for the microwave.

Reflection Questions

1. Have you ever made a similar mistake? If so, how did it make you feel?
2. Would it have been considered professional negligence if the microwave error had harmed a baby? Why or why not?

A Lunch We'll Never Forget

We routinely ordered out when working in the NICU. You learn quickly who delivers and the hours they deliver. On nights, we knew which restaurants would deliver the latest. We also knew our own coffee shop only stayed open until 10:00 p.m., so if you wanted something, you had to order it before then. Additionally, our cafeteria closed at 8:00 p.m.

On this specific day, the weather was nice, and we decided to have one of the nurses walk to the local sandwich shop, which was just down the street, to get us all lunch. Several of us ordered that day. I know that because I also know several of us were sick later that day—very sick. We all ate our lunch on rotating shifts and got back to work. As the afternoon progressed, several of us started feeling "off," specifically our stomachs.

We had one single-stall staff bathroom directly outside of the NICU. If that bathroom were occupied, you would have to go to the public bathrooms in the hallway. I paint this picture because, unfortunately, there were several of us who needed to use the bathroom in an emergency fashion. It was as if an alarm clock went off in our intestines, all at the same time. There was not enough deodorizing spray to cover up the destruction occurring in our tiny bathroom. It was *so* bad.

The nurses who didn't get sick had to take over caring for the babies we all were assigned to. Luckily, it was close to change of shift. I remember giving shift report from the bathroom because getting up simply was not an option. And I was the lucky one who got to use our staff bathroom. The other nurses who were sick had to use the bathrooms in the hallway. It was a grim situation, to say the least. My insides were violently escaping my body, and if I left the toilet, Heaven help us all. I remember staying in that bathroom for at least an hour after my shift. I had even slid my badge under the door so another nurse could clock me out. Clearly, I shouldn't have been getting paid for what I was doing.

When there seemed to be nothing left inside, I could drive home. However, I was sick for several days after that. We called our local health department, and they went to inspect the sandwich shop. What they found was nothing short of disturbing. Apparently, one of the workers was unwrapping the meat and placing it in the bins with his bare hands, which also had open sores on them. They offered us each a gift card to come back. Um, no thanks. To this day, I have not eaten there again, nor will I.

As I reflect back on that time, I laugh. But I certainly was not laughing that day. I also realized you haven't truly given a good report until you have given it from a bathroom stall—yet another reason why it is important for nurses to keep up with their charting.

Reflection Questions

1. What if, while in the bathroom, something would have happened to one of the babies she was caring for? Would Valerie have been responsible?
2. Consider what might have happened if every nurse working that shift had gotten food poisoning. How do you think they would have handled that?

The Surprise of a Simple Touch

To start off this story, I want to set the scene for readers that I am easily startled. If I see a bug I am not expecting, I scream, and Heaven forbid it actually touches me. I have been this way my entire life. My mom told me a story about when I was 2 years old, in the back of the car, and started screaming and crying, and they had no idea why. Apparently, a fly landed on me. Once they removed the fly, I settled down. To this day, I am still just as ridiculous. I once jumped out of a moving vehicle I was driving (luckily, going at a slow speed) because of a spider crawling on the seat. Or if someone comes into a room and I wasn't expecting them, I scream. It is what it is.

With that said, we had a baby in the NICU whose lower arm, wrist, and hand hadn't fully developed. The arm was shorter as well, and at the end of it, where the wrist should start, were two soft pieces of cartilage, which looked a bit like a claw. He never moved that arm, so the other nurses and I assumed he couldn't. One night, when my arm was inside the isolette, the baby moved that arm for the first time and softly pinched me. The sudden unexpected contact took me so off guard that I screamed and yanked my arm out of the isolette. Everyone turned to stare, wondering what had happened. What was so egregious that caused me to scream? The simple touch of a sweet baby boy. Once I got it back together, everyone was laughing at me, and I, too, couldn't stop laughing.

I think back and wonder if his soft pinch on my arm was him simply reaching out to say hello. Maybe I was his favorite nurse, and he told me in his own special way. Either way, nursing is a serious job, but sometimes you just have to laugh, even at yourself. I hope never to be so serious that I can't laugh at the little things, including myself. Because if you know me, you know there's lots to laugh about.

Reflection Questions

1. What are your initial thoughts when reading this story?
2. Think back to a time when you simply had to laugh at yourself. How did that make you feel?

Stop Squirting Me!

We used to have these pink saline "bullets" that held 1–2 ml of saline. Sometimes when we were bored or just feeling mischievous, we would take them and squirt them on each other. When we moved into the new NICU, we were in pods, and you could take the saline bullet and squirt it up and over the pod—to add an extra element of surprise. Those were the best times: when you could really surprise someone and when it was hard for them to tell who had done it or where it came from. One night, though, it all came back to bite me because one of the nurses, instead of squirting me with the saline bullet, filled up a 60 ml syringe and then squirted it on me, making it look like I had peed my scrubs. Luckily, we wore hospital scrubs, so I could just change my scrubs. Every time I see those pink bullets of saline, I stop and smile. Silly nurse, those aren't supposed to be used to loosen up respiratory secretions; those are to squirt each other with. Perhaps the manufacturer should sell them under a different type of label.

Reflection Questions

1. Think back to a time when you used something at work or home for a completely different purpose than what it was intended for. How did it make you feel to know you invented a new usage for the item?
2. What were your thoughts when you read about the nurses squirting saline on each other?

Grandma, Put Down the Baby

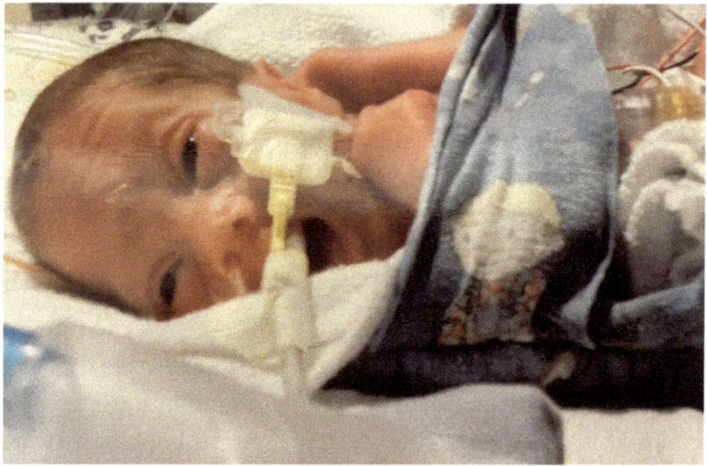

IMG 4.1

My cousin Lyle was in the NICU because he was born at 24 weeks, so he spent quite a bit of time in the NICU, and thus so did my family. I'd have to say it was really weird having my family be where I worked. There is home and work life, and they had rarely mixed until this time. My grandmother would frequently visit, and one day I caught her picking up another crying baby, trying to get it to stop crying. I had to explain that she could not just pick up other babies, that she had to stay by Lyle's bedside and that technically, she couldn't pick him up unless one of the nurses was there. She looked at me like I had three heads and said, "But the baby was crying." To that, I replied, "Yes, I know, grandma, but you just can't pick up other babies—even if they are crying. It is an infection control thing. I understand why you want to do it; you just can't." Even after that day, I would catch her around the NICU giving babies their pacifiers or just talking to other babies. The nurses would come and tell me, "You need to control your grandma." I was like, "Clearly, I can't." I'll never forget the charge nurse saying, "Blanche, you cannot touch the other babies. If you keep doing it, we won't let you come see Lyle." The look my grandma gave that nurse was priceless. The good news is that my cousin did really well in the NICU and eventually went home, and grandma finally stopped messing with the other babies, which was almost worse because she would come to tell me about it and expect me to fix it. God love her. As a side note, most 24-week babies have lifelong concerns after being born at that gestation, but by the grace of God, Lyle is a thriving teenager now whose favorite subject in school is "dodgeball."

Reflection Questions

1. Imagine yourself in a similar situation. How might you have replied to your grandma?
2. What are the reasons Valerie's grandma can't touch the other babies?

Flying Poop and Pee

When changing a baby's diapers, you never know what might happen. To get an idea of the scenario, isolettes have holes in each end, as well as holes for your arms to go into. Sometimes the holes at the end are open, and sometimes they are closed. In this specific situation, they were open. As I was changing the baby's diaper, they pooped, and not just any poop: projectile poop directly out the side hole of the isolette and onto the next baby's crib. Luckily, we cover the top of all cribs with blankets to shield the light; otherwise, the poop would have been all over the other baby. As it was, the poop was all over the crib and blankets. It was quite a mess.

On a different occasion, I changed a little boy's diaper. When the diaper was off, he started to pee—a straight stream directly up—and unfortunately, his mouth was open at the exact same time because he was crying, so the pee went directly into his mouth. It was as if it was happening in slow motion, but there wasn't anything I could do about it. Needless to say, that was an interesting one to document in the chart. The number of pee and poo stories I have is innumerable, but these are two of my favorites.

Reflection Questions

1. If you were the nurse, how would you have documented the urine "situation"?
2. Think back to a pee and/or poo story in your life. How did you respond?

The Tornado Is Coming!

I have always been afraid of tornados. In fact, I don't remember a time I wasn't afraid of them. This fear likely stems from the time when a tornado hit the grade school I attended on one of my first days of kindergarten. I remember hearing windows breaking and kids screaming. I specifically remember an older boy who was crying, and I remember thinking to myself, "If he is scared, we are all goners." Nobody was hurt, but it certainly left a lasting impression in my mind.

Fast-forward to one of the days I was working as a nurse in the NICU. We knew about the tornado watch, but we never did anything until it became a warning. Then came the warning and the sirens. Super. We had several babies on ventilators and not enough portable oxygen tanks, so some had to stay in the NICU while the others went to a more centralized and safer location. You see, we were on the concourse, and the length of the NICU unit was filled with windows. Windows are nice for letting the sun in but not so nice when the tornado sirens are going off.

As the charge nurse, I stayed back with another nurse and a respiratory therapist. We covered the babies in bath blankets and then attempted to cover the windows with bath blankets. I was the smallest one, so I stood up on the counters behind the beds to tape the blankets to the windows, and regardless of how much tape I used, they wouldn't stay. I could feel myself beginning to panic. I thought to myself, "This is how I am going to die." I was to the point of hyperventilation when I told the security guard who was helping us, "So, this is what is going to save us? A bath blanket that won't stay taped to the window?"

He could see I was losing it, and with the straightest face, replied, "Valerie, tornados don't hit hospitals, ever. It's because of the fan they have on the top of the building. The fan deters the tornado and ultimately prevents it from hitting the hospital." I remember replying, "Really?!?!" He replied, "Yes, we just do this as a precaution, but it's impossible for the hospital to get hit." I was so relieved. I had no idea. Why didn't everybody have this magical fan? I took a deep breath and got down from the counter.

I promptly told the other nurse who was with me the great news. I wasn't even done with my story before she began laughing. I asked her why she was laughing, and she replied, "Valerie, you are so gullible. There is no fan. He made that up to get you to stop freaking out. Honestly, we're in the concourse, so we'll be the first to go." I am confident that the look on my face was priceless. I preferred the security officer's version of the story. I joked around with him for lying, but honestly, he probably did the best thing for me. After that day, when I would see him around the hospital, we would joke about the hypothetical fan at the top of the hospital and laugh. And for anyone who might be as gullible as me, there is no fan.

Reflection Questions

1. If you were the charge nurse, how might you have responded to the tornado warning?
2. Reflect on this situation but in a more serious fashion. Is it the nurse's responsibility to stay with their patients, even if it means they themselves could die?
3. Where does the responsibility of caring for patients end for a nurse, or does it?
4. The security guard told a lie to calm Valerie down. Do you think this was the right thing to do? Why, or why not?

PART V

Unforgettable NICU Stories

Just 5 More Minutes

We were called to a scheduled C-section of a mom with placental accreta. Placental accreta is a high-risk pregnancy complication where the placenta attaches too deeply to the uterine wall. There are different types of placental accreta, and this mom specifically had placenta percreta, which meant that the placenta had grown through the uterus into the surrounding organs—in her case, her bladder and intestines. The C-section was being held in the main operating room (OR) to accommodate the large team of surgeons attending the delivery. Before the delivery, the mom was told that due to the extensiveness of the placental accreta, she only had a 50% chance of surviving the delivery. They had also decided to do the delivery at 30 weeks because the risk to the baby was greater if she stayed inside than to be delivered early. I was the NICU RN attending the delivery.

When I got to the OR, I instantly noticed people everywhere. There were different teams assigned to different stages of the delivery. There were also bags of blood hanging on poles—more than I had ever seen. The infant warmer was set up close to the mom, so I could hear everything.

As the anesthesiologist was getting ready to put the mask over the mom's face to "put her to sleep," the mom looked up at him and asked for *5 more minutes*. Then she began to cry. The anesthesiologist told her they needed to start the surgery, and the mom then started begging him to wait, crying out that she "wasn't ready to die." I can still hear her begging not to do it as he put the mask over her face and she "fell asleep" from the anesthesia. I literally could not imagine being in her place: being told that I only had a 50% chance of survival. I fought back tears until I just couldn't anymore. I still remember the feeling of the tears falling into the surgical mask.

Once the surgery started, it was nothing less than a disaster. Blood was *everywhere*, surgeons were yelling, and then the baby was finally born, and they handed her to me, and she was a pale blue color and limp. When I got her to the warmer, the neonatologist and I started the initial steps for neonatal resuscitation and quickly realized that the baby didn't have a heartbeat and wasn't breathing. We followed the initial steps (positioning the head, clearing the airway, drying the baby, removing wet linens, and stimulating the baby to breathe), but still, nothing.

After doing the initial steps of neonatal resuscitation, we transitioned to the next steps, which were assisted ventilation and then chest compressions. I remember thinking how the mom thought she might die, but never once did she think her baby would. We finally got a heartbeat and needed to transfer the baby to the NICU so that we could continue caring for her.

Meanwhile, the mom's surgery was not going well. I remember pushing the transporter over puddles of blood on the floor (Reason 758 why you never wear your nursing shoes in your house). I had seen many things, but never anything like this. I heard them shouting, "We're losing her" as we walked out. I left the OR with the assumption that the mom would not survive.

Once in the NICU, we were able to give the baby transfusions, and along with other medications and assisted ventilation, we were able to stabilize her. The dad was able to come in and visit, and I remember him asking how his wife was doing, but I honestly had no idea what to say, so I said, "My focus was on your daughter, but I know that the surgical team is going to do everything they can to care for your wife." This was not a lie. I knew they were doing everything they could. I just wasn't sure if it would be enough.

I went home that night not knowing if the mom survived, as she was still in the OR. The next morning when I came to work, I was scrubbing in at the sinks (we had to scrub in/sanitize our hands and arms before every shift), and next to me at the other sink was a mom, scrubbing in to see her baby for the first time. She was still in a hospital bed. I quickly realized it was the mom from the delivery the day prior. She had lived!

I was scrubbing my hands, and tears of joy streamed down my face. I tried blowing it off, like my eyes were watering because of allergies, but it was clear I was making it up and that they were real tears. Thankfully, they were tears of joy and relief. I was assigned to the same baby and got to hand her to the mom to hold for the first time. I explained to the mom that I was the nurse in the delivery the day before. She looked me in the eyes and tearfully said, "Thank you for everything." Both mom and baby did well and eventually were discharged home.

To this day, I can instantly be transported back to that OR suite and can hear the mom begging for her life. I can hear the surgeons yelling. I see multiple bags of blood hanging on poles and blood all over the floor. However, I also see the miracle of the mom holding her daughter for the first time and the looks on their faces when we placed the baby in the car seat, and they drove home—with everyone alive. Not all stories end this well, but on the really bad days, I would remember this one and smile.

Reflection Questions

1. What were the hardest parts for you when reading this story?
2. How would you have managed your feelings if you were in this same situation, hearing the mom begging for "just 5 more minutes"?

Not Again!

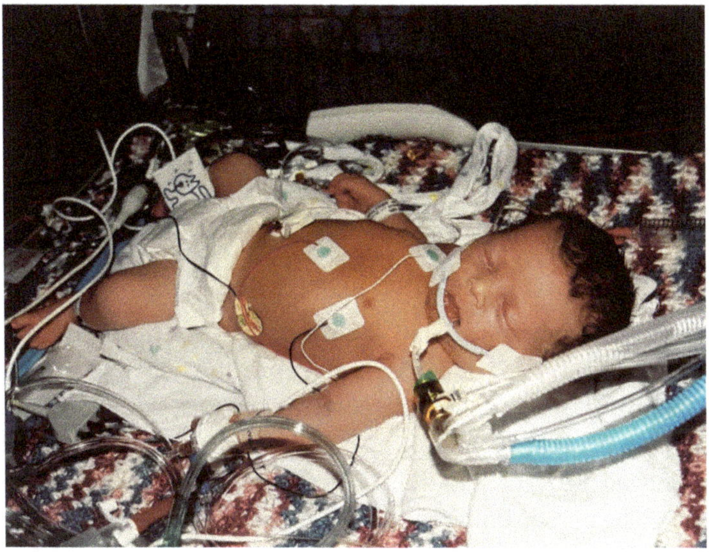

IMG 5.1

May 17, 2006, was not just another day. It was my first day back to work after being on an extended medical leave. It was my first day back to work caring for babies after my babies had died. I knew going back to the NICU would be hard, but it was all I ever knew, and I was ready to return to a sense of normalcy again. Little did I know how hard my first day would be.

The day was going pretty well, and I was initially given an easy assignment. However, we received notification that we were getting a transport admission, and since I had the "easy" assignment, I would have to take the admission. I rarely took easy assignments, so I was looking forward to the distraction until I realized the admission was going to be a Penn baby.

When Mason was 8 months old (refer to "It Wasn't Supposed to Happen" story), his parents, Tyler and Kellie, found out they were pregnant. For people who were told they wouldn't get pregnant, they sure found a way to make it happen, and this time, it was a surprise! Kellie once again found herself in preterm labor, but this time at 32 weeks. She spent 2 weeks in our hospital and was discharged home for bed rest. Kellie reminded me that when she was in our hospital, I had come in and washed her hair. It is interesting how memories work because, to this day, that is not a memory I have. However, if Kellie said I did it, I am sure I did. It absolutely sounds like something I would do. After all, clean hair is very important. After a week of bed rest, Kellie delivered her daughter, Millie, at the hospital in her hometown.

Millie couldn't be outdone by her brothers, and she, too, needed NICU care and thus was transferred to our NICU. She was stable on transport, and the admission was supposed to be fairly routine, except the Penn babies do nothing routine. She began to be less stable toward the end of the transport, and by the time I admitted her, she coded (stopped breathing and didn't have a heartbeat). I quickly moved into resuscitation mode and began doing chest compressions. The person doing compressions says, "One, and two, and three, and breathe, and one, and two, and three, and breathe," to let the resuscitation team stay in rhythm with the ventilation and compressions. I had done this more times than I would have liked, but this time was different.

As I was pressing on her chest, tears streamed down my face. It was like an out-of-body experience. My body just took over. I had done this several times, so I instinctively knew what to do. Meanwhile, my heart was ripping into a thousand pieces. Emotions came flooding back—emotions from losing Miles and from losing my twins. I thought, "If she dies, I might die. I cannot take this." All of this was going through my head in a matter of microseconds.

As if it was yesterday, I remember leaning down into the warmer, and as if Millie could understand me, I told her, "You can't do this. I'm not strong enough. You must live." I kept saying it over and over. One of the other nurses could see I was not handling the situation well and stepped in to do the resuscitation for me. I stood and watched while I prayed and cried. By the Grace of God, she pulled out of it. We got her back. Just then, her dad called to check on her, and they handed the phone to me. I didn't even try to fake it. He already knew. I told him as objectively as possible what had happened and that she was stable now.

Millie made a full recovery and was discharged home in record time. I remember seeing her in her car seat, getting ready to go home. With tears in my eyes, I thanked God for her recovery. She is now a beautiful and thriving teenager. After that, the Penns decided not to have any more biological children (thank God because I'm not sure I could take it again). They adopted a spunky little boy, Madden, from South Korea.

As nurses, we are told not to get attached to patients and their families. Well, I certainly broke that rule. My life story has been uniquely interwoven with the life of the Penn family, so much so that in 2008, Tyler officiated my husband and I's wedding. To this day, we are still very good friends. I was there for them during some of the darkest moments of their lives, and they were there for me too. It has been a privilege to watch Mason, Millie, and Madden grow up through the years. Sometimes, when you know how to follow the rules, you also know how to break them. If I had to do it over, I would do the same thing all over again.

Reflection Questions

1. What do you think about the "unspoken" rule of nurses not getting attached to their patients/families?
2. If you got especially attached to a certain baby, would you want to be their primary caregiver or would you be scared to be overly involved?
3. Imagine yourself giving chest compressions to a baby. How does that make you feel?

Don't Ask for Anything

We had a unit secretary in our NICU who wasn't always the friendliest. In fact, I was told when I started specifically not to ask her for anything. Except, it makes life hard for a nurse not to be able to ask for assistance from the support staff, especially the secretary. Nurses were literally afraid of her, and I'm not going to lie: I was too.

One day, we needed to order more needles, and guess whose job it is to order needles? The unit secretary! So, the nurses were trying to figure out how to do it themselves so they didn't have to bother her, which I thought was crazy. So, I took the package the needles came in and wrote a nice note asking her to reorder these for us, please. I even put a smiley face on the note and then left it on her keyboard. As soon as she saw it, she came into the NICU and asked in a loud and accusatory tone who put the note on her keyboard. As if in unison, all the nurses pointed at me. Thanks a lot, guys. She then stomped into the NICU and yelled at me for putting it on her desk. I said as kindly as possible, "I put it on your desk with the note because I was afraid to ask you to order them." She was taken aback by this and asked me why. As all the nurses stared, waiting for my response, I politely said, "Sometimes I get the feeling that you don't like me." Actually, I was pretty sure she hated all the other nurses and me.

Come to find out, she didn't hate us. She apologized for giving off that "vibe" and said she would try to do better in the future. Afterward, I would leave notes with smiley faces on her keyboard, but no more notes to order things. The entire NICU breathed a sigh of relief that day. It made me think that sometimes we don't realize how we come across until some brave soul brings it to our attention. May this story inspire you to confront the "bully" in your life. They might turn out to be your very best friend!

Reflection Questions

1. Have you ever encountered a bully? If so, how did you respond?
2. What might happen if you confronted your bully in the same way Valerie did?

You Can't Do "That" Here

I was caring for a critically ill baby whose admission meconium screening (drug test on the baby's feces) returned positive for methamphetamines, cocaine, and marijuana. The Division of Child and Family Services (DCFS) was involved in the baby's case, but the parents were still allowed to visit, which they didn't do very often.

One of the days they came to visit, they were being extra affectionate toward each other at the bedside. Normally, I wouldn't care if the parents gave each other a little hug or kiss, but this was way more than that. I had mentioned to them that their behavior was inappropriate and if they needed to be "like that," to take it outside of the NICU. So, they did. They left, and then about an hour later, they came back.

I was caring for another baby and looked over, and the dad had the mom pinned up against the isolette "aggressively" making out and, before I could get to them, had begun having sex at their baby's bedside. I mean, there are no words for the extreme inappropriateness of this. For one, their baby was critically ill. Secondly, the NICU was full of people. And lastly, having sex at your baby's hospital bedside is *never* okay. I got them to stop, letting them know you can't do "that" in the NICU, and then asked them to leave, which, thank goodness, they did.

The NICU can be an intense place, but it was extra "intense" that day. We notified DCFS, and for that along with many other reasons, the baby went into foster care. I often wonder if the parents ever got "clean" and if they ever got custody of their baby. I guess there are some things we will never know, but one thing I do know is that you can't do "that" in the NICU.

Reflection Questions

1. What are your initial feelings toward the parents of this baby?
2. Did knowing the mom tested positive for methamphetamines, cocaine, and marijuana alter your perception of her?
3. How would you manage your feelings toward the parents when caring for this baby, knowing that we treat all parents equally?

You Only Get One Orientation

When I first started in the NICU, I had a primary preceptor and a secondary preceptor. This is because I was scheduled from 7:00 a.m.–3:00 p.m. Monday through Friday for my orientation, and the nurses worked 12-hour shifts. Getting matched with the right preceptor is the difference between a good orientation and a bad orientation. And although I was a smidge scared of my primary preceptor, I knew she would be an excellent teacher.

She had worked in the NICU for several years and had a history of taking the more critical babies, which was perfect because those were my favorite babies to take. The more I worked with my primary preceptor, the less afraid I was of her. She had high standards, which I appreciated because I did too. But on days she wasn't there, I was paired with my secondary preceptor, who was completely different from my primary preceptor.

I had difficulty following my secondary preceptor. She was an amazing nurse, but her technique was completely opposite of what I was being taught by my primary preceptor. She was all over the place, and most days, I couldn't even find her. She always had her hand in something, which was extremely distracting for me. I was very rule-oriented and was comforted by meticulously following the protocols. She seemed to have her own protocols, which, if I'm honest, were really hard to navigate.

I was supposed to be on orientation for 3 months. It was only my third week, and I knew this wouldn't work. I could have gone to the manager and asked to be switched. The secondary preceptor would have never known. Sometimes the easiest thing isn't always the right thing. So, I pulled her aside and let her know how I was struggling. I told her I respected her as a nurse but that I was having a hard time learning from her. Luckily, she understood.

As a nurse, you are taught to advocate for your patients and yourself. I mustered up every ounce of bravery I had as a new nurse to advocate for myself and ask for a different preceptor. It was not easy, but I did it. I worked alongside that nurse my entire time in the NICU; in fact, she just recently retired. To this day, I am proud of myself for sticking up for what I needed and thankful that she wasn't offended. You see, you only get one orientation.

Reflection Questions

1. If you were in Valerie's shoes, would you have spoken up about your need for a different preceptor or just let it go? Regardless of your decision, why did you choose it?
2. As the nurse, what would you do if you noticed another nurse was not following a policy?

Just Say "No" to the Nap

For obvious reasons, hospitals are open 24/7, 365 days a year, which means if you choose to work in the hospital as a nurse, you, too, will work 24/7, 365 days a year. Of course, when I graduated from nursing school, I foolishly requested the day shift, which, understandably, I didn't get. I was hired onto the night shift and worked nights for almost 5 years until a day position finally came available, which I snagged and never looked back!

The night shift is not for the faint of heart. Forcing your body to stay awake when it is supposed to be sleeping is hard stuff. I would try to coordinate my schedule so that I worked several nights in a row and then had several off so I could transition from sleeping during the day to sleeping during the night, but if I'm honest, it never worked that well. If I was working three 12-hour night shifts in a row, I would do my best to sleep in the first day, then go to work and stay up all night. I'd sleep during the day the next two days, and then when my stent was over, I would only sleep till around 11:00 or 12:00 in the day and then force myself to wake up so that I could sleep that night.

Those days were the worst. You know that feeling when you are so tired you are sick to your stomach and have a terrible headache? At least for me, that's how it was. One night, for whatever reason, I didn't sleep during the day, but I had worked the night before and then had to go back to work another 12-hour night shift. It was brutal. I remember sitting out at the nurses desk begging the clock to move faster, all the while feeling like I could vomit at any second. The seconds dragged on for days, and so, on my 30-minute break, I had the fantastic idea to go sleep in the nurses lounge.

I figured I'd get in a quick cat nap and back to work I'd go, completely refreshed and ready to tackle the rest of the shift. Well, that is exactly the opposite of what happened. Of course, I fell immediately to sleep, but when my 30-minute alarm went off, I knew I had made a horrible decision. I could barely raise my head off the floor and then just had to drag myself back to work, feeling worse than I did before I laid down. Some might be able to take a quick cat nap and feel better. Some nurses might even love the night shift. But not me.

Working the night shift wasn't all negative, though. I spent more time with the babies, as there were fewer distractions. Fewer procedures were being done unless they were emergencies. Fewer people were at the bedside (rounding took place during the day, and rarely were families there at 2:00 a.m.). As a nurse, it also really solidified my skills, as there weren't as many people around, so you often just had to figure it out. We ran on bare bones, so you made it work with what you had.

We also had the opportunity to weigh the babies on nights, which was kind of fun. That was when I would clean up their bed, get them in a new outfit or snuggle up (something we used to swaddle the babies who were in isolettes and warmers when we couldn't use blankets), and then snuggle them back in for the night. So, it wasn't all bad, but a word of caution for those new to nights: Just say "no" to the nap.

Reflection Questions

1. Think back to a time when you were ridiculously tired. How did you manage the situation?
2. Would you be better off with a short cat nap or just staying up all night?
3. How might you manage your sleeping schedule if you worked the night shift?

One-Way Bus to Mexico

There was a Hispanic family who was in the area as migrant workers. The mom was 24 weeks pregnant and working in the fields when she went into labor. She was rushed by ambulance to our hospital, where she quickly delivered the perfect little 24-week baby boy. They were unfortunately here on a temporary status and, as soon as the baby was born, had to return to Mexico. Our social workers did all they could to ensure she and her husband could stay, but unfortunately, it didn't work.

I was this baby's primary nurse and vowed to do everything I could to keep the parents in the loop. I remember getting their address, and each week I would take pictures of their son in the cutest little outfits and write a letter to them. The letter was from the viewpoint of their son. I would have him "talk" about how big he was getting and how much he loved them. This was before the era of Google Translate, so my neighbor from Peru, Nathalie, would translate the letters from English to Spanish, and I would mail them off, sealing the back of the envelope with his tiny footprints.

As time passed and he was closer to going home, we weren't sure how it would all work out. What our social work team planned out is that the dad was going to come back, as he had a visa to come to the United States. They had very little money, so we decided to pull together money to purchase a bus ticket for him and the baby to go back to Mexico.

We knew they didn't have any supplies, so in addition to the bus ticket, we got together all of the supplies they needed to care for their son, including a car seat. We even bought suitcases to put the supplies in. We had to be mindful not to buy too much because it was just the dad coming and he would have to transport everything back himself, including his son.

I still remember the day the dad came to get his son. When I handed him his son to hold for the first time, he cried. I cried. Anyone in the near vicinity was crying. It was a super emotional time. I remember him leaving the NICU, his son in one hand, suitcase in the other, and a one-way ticket to Mexico. I smiled as they left, thinking about how elated his mom would be when they were finally all reunited.

Reflection Questions

1. How did it make you feel when you read that the family had to return to Mexico?
2. Imagine yourself in the mother's shoes, knowing your baby is critically ill, thousands of miles away, and you cannot see them. What emotions does this bring up for you?

Permanently Grounded

After working in the NICU for some time, I joined the transport team. We were a Level III NICU and would travel to surrounding towns to transport their babies to our higher level of care. The fact that I was on the transport team was a miracle in and of itself, as I get extremely motion sick. And if you have ever been in the back of an ambulance going down the road, you know of the extreme motion occurring in the back. But, somehow, I did it. I actually loved it. I only ever got sick once, and luckily it was on the way back, and the baby was stable—not too shabby.

Then came the helicopter, which was quite an upgrade for our hospital and our NICU. We were elated to have the opportunity to get to our surrounding hospitals quicker, and what better way than via air? The NICU manager at the time had asked me to be the lead transport nurse for our flight team, and I excitedly said yes! You see, size and weight are key factors in the helicopter, and I met both criteria. I also had the experience of managing critical babies on transport. There was just one catch, my stomach.

We decided it might be best to do a test flight, especially with my history of motion sickness. So, I got all buckled in, and we headed off for the test flight. I would like to say it went well, but that is not the case. In fact, I started throwing up, and I could still see our hospital. It took less than 5 minutes for my stomach to say, "No thanks!" Here's the deal: I am not a "pretty puker." There are people who can vomit and then just go about their day—not me. I look like death, and there is zero way anyone would sign consent for me to take their baby looking, myself, like death. Test flight number one failed.

This ruined many plans for our NICU, so the manager asked me to try again, but this time taking medication to help with motion sickness. I knew I couldn't take regular Dramamine, as it knocked me out, so I picked up some nondrowsy Dramamine, and off I went. We only had 15 minutes from the time of the call until when we were supposed to be in the air, so I took the nondrowsy Dramamine and, 15 minutes later, got in the helicopter. This time I lasted 10 minutes before I started vomiting.

The manager was patiently waiting for me to return with good news. Nope. I went straight to her office after getting off the helicopter. It was lunchtime. She was eating a fish sandwich. She didn't even get out the full sentence of asking how it went, and I vomited again in her trash can. I suppose that's your answer. She wasn't happy, and honestly, neither was I. I was so excited to be on our flight team, but my stomach had different plans—plans that required me to be permanently grounded.

Reflection Questions

1. What is the first thing that comes to mind when you think about flight nursing? Would you want to do it?
2. How might you react if you were on a transport, in charge of a critically ill baby, and got physically ill from motion sickness?

Denial Is a Powerful Thing

We were called to a vaginal delivery of unknown gestational age. The mom was admitted to the emergency department (ED) with complaints of stomach pain, thinking it was appendicitis. The staff in the ED quickly realized it was not her appendix but rather that she was having a baby. She was crowning as they rapidly pushed her in a wheelchair from the ED to L&D. Crowning means that the baby's head has become visible in the birth canal. It won't be long before the baby is born.

When I got into the delivery room, I saw that the baby was crowning, and the mom was yelling at the obstetrician to stop "touching her down there." She reiterated more than once that she wasn't having a baby, that there was no way she was pregnant, and that her appendix was causing the issues. I couldn't believe what I was hearing. She refused to push, but somehow the baby was born, a perfect full-term precious baby girl. Once the baby was born, they brought her over to me, where I completed the initial steps of neonatal resuscitation. The baby was doing great, but I heard the mom say, "That's not my baby." I couldn't believe what I was hearing. This baby clearly just came from her body. She started screaming at us that the baby wasn't hers and to get it out of the room. So, we got a crib and took the baby to the newborn nursery.

I found out later that she had signed over her rights to the baby and went home later that day. This sweet baby girl was in our newborn nursery for 7 days before a very lucky adoptive family came to pick her up. In the meantime, I hated that she didn't have a name, so I named her Emily. To this day, I have no idea if her family kept that name, but for at least a week, she was baby girl Emily. I always knew denial was powerful; I just had no idea how powerful it could be.

Reflection Questions

1. As you read this story, specifically the part about how the mom said, "That's not my baby," how did that make you feel?
2. Imagine yourself in that delivery room. How might you have responded to the mother?
3. Why do you think Valerie gave the baby a name? Do you think it is a good idea?

Every Little Girl Deserves a Bow

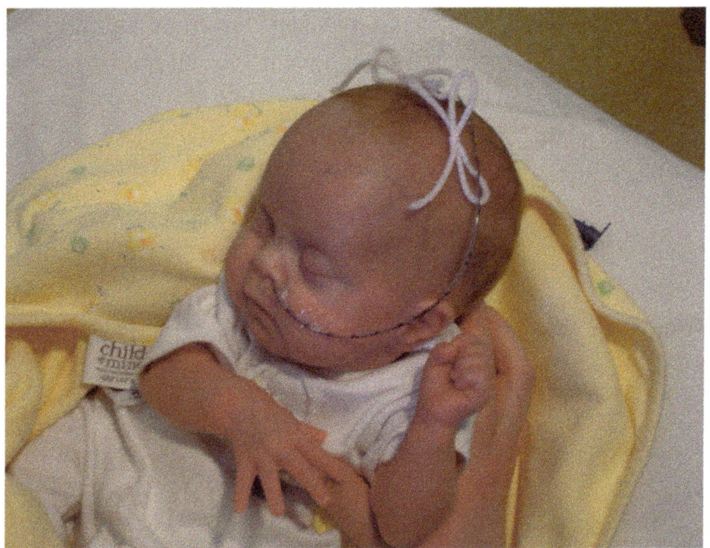

IMG 5.2

When working in the NICU, we would often get updates on the moms in the antepartum unit. These were moms who were pregnant but not stable. They required some sort of hospital intervention, like monitoring for contractions, receiving antibiotics, among several other potential reasons. One mom was admitted to L&D at 18 weeks, as her "bag of water" had broken. This is a normal process for someone around 40 weeks gestation but not 18 weeks. In fact, the likelihood of this mom making it to viability (24 weeks) would be slim to none. However, we should always try, and try is what they did.

This specific mom's name is Charity, and her husband's name is Joshua. I am still in contact with them, even though I rarely cared for their daughter, Cydney. This is because Cydney was born at 27½ weeks on January 18, 2005, just a day before Miles and Mason were born. And as you know from reading their story, they required much care, especially sweet baby Miles.

I now have the opportunity to watch Cydney grow up. I see pictures of her on Facebook, and each time I do, I thank God for the miracle of her life. She is a thriving teenage girl in cheerleading and other activities, all of which we never thought would have been possible. But God had different plans.

When gathering information for this book, I talked to Cydney's mom. I hadn't ever told her this, but I, along with many other NICU nurses, prayed for her when she was on the antepartum unit. No mom had made it as long as Charity did, and we were really rooting for her. What seemed impossible was slowly becoming possible, week after week that Cydney stayed "inside." Although I wasn't one of Cydney's primary nurses, I did make a small difference in her life, specifically with pink bows I would put in her hair.

You see, having to witness your baby fight for their life in the NICU is unimaginable, and so I wanted to bring a little bit of normalcy to their fight in the way of a pink bow. It was a skill I had acquired over the years, a skill I wasn't taught in nursing school but still a very important skill. Even for those little girls with hardly any hair, I could still make it happen. And if they happened to be born with no hair, no problem at all. My secret was a tiny dab of Vaseline under the bow, which helped it to stick like a charm, or at least until the photos were taken.

You see, because every little girl deserves a bow.

Reflection Questions

1. What impact do you think the pink bows might have had on the families of the babies in the NICU?
2. What other "skills" have you witnessed in nurses that were not skills they would have learned in nursing school?

Watch Out!

We received a call from L&D that they were going to be delivering 26-week triplets. A 26-week single admission is a lot, but for triplets, we were going to need to call in extra help. Each of those babies would need its own nurse at the delivery and, initially, a one-on-one nurse for their admission. I suppose I am trying to set the scene for the reader that these types of admissions were nothing short of organized chaos.

I was the charge nurse, and after calling in our on-call nurse and begging a few others to come in, we were as ready as we could be. I stayed back in the NICU to get the beds ready and then was available to help with the admissions. The babies did well in the OR and then, one by one, came to the NICU in their transport isolettes.

Luckily, we don't have to take the babies to radiology for general x-rays, as they have a portable machine that can come to us. Each of the babies had an arterial line placed, and radiology was on their way to come to take films to check placement. The portable x-ray machine is huge. It almost reminded me of a small Zamboni. It also had a moving "arm" on the top that would fit over our warmers to take the x-ray.

Typically, they don't move the arm out from the machine until they are ready for the film. They especially don't lock it in place until everything is perfect—except on this day. Of course, I wasn't paying any attention and was expecting things to be like they always were. I turned around from the baby's warmer to give the radiology tech room to put the machine, and he already had the arm out and locked but between the beds and right at eye level to me.

This meant that as I turned around, with quite a bit of "oomph," I smashed right into it with the side of my face. Simultaneously as I was turning, the tech said, "Watch out!" but it was too late. I hit it so hard that I immediately fell to the floor. Clearly, there is a piece of time I don't remember, but when I came to, there was a level of panic in the NICU that was palpable, and wow, did my head hurt! It quickly swelled around the temple area and looked as if I was growing another head.

Our emergency department was backed up, and because I felt fine, other than the terrible headache, I decided to just go home. Once I was home, I started throwing up, and the pain worsened. I didn't want to return to the hospital, so I took a pill to help me sleep (*very* bad idea) and went to bed. The next day I had a black eye, the swelling hadn't decreased much, and the pain was still there.

The hospital had me come back in, and they did x-rays of my face and skull. Nothing was broken except for maybe my ego, so I went home on concussion protocol and sucked it up. My eye was black for days, and it took forever for the "second head" to go away. After that, when I would see the x-ray machine, I would give it *plenty* of distance between the machine and myself. The tech, who I was friends with, later showed me the arm of the machine I had hit, and there was a part of it that was bent, compliments of my head. For those who know me well, this type of accident would only happen to me. The common phrase is, "If it's going to happen to anybody, it's going to happen to Valerie." And they aren't far off.

Reflection Questions

1. If you were in Valerie's shoes after the x-ray accident, what would you have done?
2. Why was her going home and taking a sleeping pill a bad idea?
3. As the charge nurse, how would you manage the admission of three critical babies at the same time?

The Dreaded Snowstorm

One winter, when I was working at the NICU, there was a forecasted snowstorm that was expected to leave roads unpassable. Warnings had gone out to stay at home, as travel was dangerous, if not impossible. Many businesses were shut down, but for obvious reasons, the hospitals must stay open, and for them to stay open, staff, including nurses, must be there.

I was scheduled to work the first night of the storm but then had the following 3 days off. The hospital offered incentives for nurses to stay the night to ensure proper staffing due to the storm. I was one of the nurses who agreed to stay, and honestly, I didn't really have a choice because since I lived out of town, there was no way I could have made it back home.

That night, the house officer was working on assigning rooms for the nurses to sleep in. The nurses who had been at the hospital for several years began talking about the "haunted" floor—just what you want to hear when you are going to have to stay on said haunted floor. They said there was a rumor that the call lights would go off in rooms with no patients. The unit had been shut down for renovations, and yet still, the call lights would go off. They said the construction crew refused to be there after dark. I had no idea if they were just messing with me or not, but wasn't really interested in finding out.

I patiently awaited my room assignment only to find out it was on the haunted floor. Lovely. I tried bargaining my way to a different floor, but there were no other options. I even contemplated revoking my decision to stay, which honestly wasn't even an option, as there was no way I could have gone home. So, with all my courage, I walked to my assigned bed after my shift. I cracked open the door and thought I saw someone in the bed. Okay, Valerie, this is your mind playing tricks on you, as the nurses had said that staff would even see patients in the beds who weren't actually there. So, I walked into the room, and guess what? There *was* someone in the bed. I screamed. He screamed, and I ran as fast as I could down the hall and ultimately back to the NICU. I called the house officer and told them about the incident. They apologized, as they didn't realize a medical resident had also been assigned to that room. I wonder if the resident knew about the haunted floor stories and if he could fall back to sleep after I woke him with my blood-curdling scream. I didn't care. I wasn't going back.

I had previously worked on the postpartum unit and knew that the room at the end of the hallway was rarely occupied and so asked about that room. Luckily, it was available, and they agreed to let me sleep there. I felt so much more comfortable in that room, but still moved the sofa and the dresser in front of the door. I didn't get much sleep, but at least I wasn't on the haunted floor. I ended up taking on two additional shifts, which meant I had to sleep there for 2 days. The next day got a little easier but still wasn't good.

Before becoming a nurse, I never considered that nurses and other hospital staff might have to stay at the hospital during times of bad weather. It was just part of the job. Somebody has to take care of the patients. There are, unfortunately, no snow days for healthcare workers. I even remember the hospital working with local plowing companies to go and get nurses who were scheduled to work if they couldn't get there themselves. Way to think outside the box! As I continued on in my career, there were other times I stayed at the hospital, but none were quite as memorable as this time.

Reflection Questions

1. Would you have been scared to stay on the haunted floor?
2. Can you think of any other jobs that require workers 24/7, 365 days a year, regardless of the weather?

Precepting Fail

When we had new nurses start, I was often one of the preceptors. I loved teaching, which is also part of the reason I went back to school and got my master's degree and, ultimately, my DNP (doctor of nursing practice). I remember a time when I was the charge nurse and realized that I had precepted every nurse on the shift with me. It was a pretty cool feeling to know that I had trained everyone there, and although I am confident their memories aren't all "kittens and rainbows," they did learn the "right" way. It was important that we followed all of the procedures as they were written. It was also important that the bedsides were cleaned, as well as the babies. And if they were a baby girl, they had a bow in their hair.

We had several nurses start at the same time, and I had the opportunity to precept a few of them. After they were off orientation, I found out that they would wait until I had filled in my schedule and then fill in their days, opposite of mine. I was horrified when I realized this. Why? One brave soul told me it was because she didn't think she could live up to my "standard," that I wanted everything to be perfect, and she didn't want to let me down. Talk about a blind spot. I had *no* idea I was inadvertently putting this much pressure on them. Moving forward, I tried to be better, but still would not compromise when it came to the babies' care.

I remember one nurse in particular. Her name is Kim. Kim was more on the quiet side, completely opposite of me, but she was a really good nurse. When she first started, though, she never left my side. She would follow me everywhere and really struggled to do anything independently. One day, I was walking to the bathroom, and she was following me. I remember telling her, "There's nothing I'm going to teach you in here," and we both laughed. After that, we had a heart-to-heart about how she needed to start doing things independently. She was far along enough in her training, and I trusted her abilities. In hindsight, I pushed her too far.

Our old NICU was set up in one long room, so if you had the bed in the first space, you could see all the beds down the row. I was caring for a baby in an isolette when I glanced down the row and saw Kim getting a micro preemie out of the isolette for the mom to hold all by herself. This baby was intubated, which alone is not a big deal. But the endotracheal tube isn't "in" very far, and sometimes the difference of half of a centimeter is the difference between it being "in" versus being out. This baby also had an umbilical arterial line, and if it was pulled too hard and came out, we would have a very bloody emergency on our hands. These babies require two to three staff to assist with the transfer from the isolette to the mom's chest for skin-to-skin holding, regardless of how many years you have been working there.

So, I see Kim pulling this baby out of the isolette all by herself. I could see the endotracheal tube and the arterial line pulling, and as if in slow motion, but also as fast as I could, went to the bedside to help. Of course, I wanted to scream, "What are you doing?!" But I couldn't. The mom was right there. So, with my best poker face, I offered my assistance, and we safely transferred the baby from the isolette to the mom's chest. Afterward, and when out of earshot of the mom, I asked Kim what she was doing. She replied, "You told me to do more things independently, so I did." I took a deep breath and explained that there are some things you can never do independently. I asked, "How is it one moment you are following me to the bathroom, and the next moment you are doing a two-assist transfer independently? Could we maybe meet in the middle?" We still joke about it to this day, but it was a great lesson for me in ensuring I gave clear direction to the nurses I was precepting but also wasn't scary in doing so. Probably if you were to ask the nurses I precepted, they would agree on the "clear direction" part, but the "less scary" part is probably debatable.

Reflection Questions

1. Reflect on how you might have responded when Kim got the critically ill baby out by herself. Do you think you would have been able to control your tone so as not to frighten the mother?
2. As a preceptor, what is your responsibility, specifically related to mistakes your preceptee might make?
3. Have you ever been in the position of training someone? What did you find difficult about this? What did you find rewarding?

Watch Out for Vacuums!

One role of a NICU nurse is the delivery nurse role. At the hospital where I worked, NICU nurses would be called to any high-risk and all C-section deliveries. As the assigned delivery nurse, I was attending a routine C-section delivery. I was standing next to the mom who was having the surgery, ready to take the baby from the obstetrician. The MD was having a hard time getting the baby out. In my mind, I thought, just cut the hole in the uterus bigger. It seemed like a logical solution to me. But I am not a surgeon. The MD asked the circulating RN for the vacuum. Now I am really questioning this and not understanding why they don't just cut the hole in the uterus bigger. Clearly, this was not the time or place to ask.

If you don't know, this is how a vacuum works. The provider will place the suction on the baby's head, and the nurse will activate the vacuum. The provider then pulls the baby out with the assistance of the vacuum. I have seen plenty of vacuums used in vaginal births but none in a C-section. Either way, they were using one on this day. As I was standing next to the OR bed, the vacuum popped off the baby's head and then splashed blood and amniotic fluid all over me—specifically, all over my face. Then the baby was born, and the MD handed them to me.

I brought the baby over to the warmer and began the initial steps of neonatal resuscitation. The baby was not doing well, and although we had done the initial steps, they still needed further interventions. As I began chest compressions, I wiped the fluid away from my eyes. Despite having a mask on, I still remember the blood and amniotic fluid running into my mouth. If I wasn't so focused on the baby's resuscitation, I think I would have been vomiting. I can still taste it in my mouth. So. Gross.

Luckily, we got the baby to come around, and after a short admission to the NICU, they were discharged home. Because I had been exposed to blood in the OR, I wrote out a hospital incident report. The mom was then tested for bloodborne pathogens. I was also tested right after the incident. Because the mom was negative (and I was too), I did not have to be retested. These are things you don't often think about. However, there are hazards when working as a nurse, some of which could be life-threatening.

Reflection Questions

1. What are other hazards nurses might face when caring for their patients?
2. Imagine having blood and amniotic fluid run down your face and into your mouth. How might you have reacted?

Never Let the Baby Die in the Bed

When I worked in the NICU, I had a policy to *never* let the baby die in the bed. There were times I was in a delivery, and the baby was dying, and the parents didn't want to hold the baby. And you know what, that was okay. Sometimes holding a baby as they die is just too much to handle as a parent. But I always felt like what was never okay was just to let them die in the bed—alone. Of course, if the parents didn't want me to hold their baby, I would have respected their decision. Luckily, this never happened.

I precepted many nurses, and if you were one of them, you would remember this strict policy. So, if a baby was dying and either the family wasn't there or they just couldn't do it, I did it. I held the precious baby in my arms as they took their last breath. If no family was there, I would softly whisper to them that they were going to be okay. They were loved. Their life mattered, and soon they would be in the arms of Jesus. And it was only after I felt them take their last breath and their tiny heart was no longer beating that I placed them back in the bed.

I give this introduction as an explanation of the following story. One of the babies I was taking care of was critically ill and actively dying. The parents were at the bedside and the mom was holding her son skin to skin. Our neonatologist had come to the bedside to give the parents an update. The decision (collaboratively with the providers and parents) had already been made not to do any resuscitation efforts. The provider gave the parents the current status of their son, none of which was good, except at the end, he said, "His blood pressure is still fairly stable."

The parents had no further questions, and the provider returned to his office. Meanwhile, the mom said to me, "I'm ready to put him back in bed to rest." I was speechless. I honestly didn't know what to say. However, I knew that the baby only had moments left to live. I had unfortunately seen this process too many times, so I knew how it typically went. And yes, the provider was right; the blood pressure was fairly stable, as the blood pressure seemed typically to be the last thing that lowered before they passed away.

I thought about it and then said as kindly and calmly as possible, "Your son is dying. You can choose to hold him while he takes his last breaths, or you can put him back in his bed. But if that happens, he will die in the bed." I was then trying to quickly figure out what I would do if she chose the latter because I don't allow babies to die in the bed. Luckily, she chose to hold him. And so, just a few minutes later, surrounded by family, that little boy died in his mother's arms.

Reflection Questions

1. How might you have responded when the mom told you she was ready to put her son back in bed?
2. Right or wrong, Valerie's "policy" was to never let a baby die in their bed. What are your thoughts on this?
3. How might you support a family who doesn't want to hold their baby while they die?

Won't You Be My Nanny?

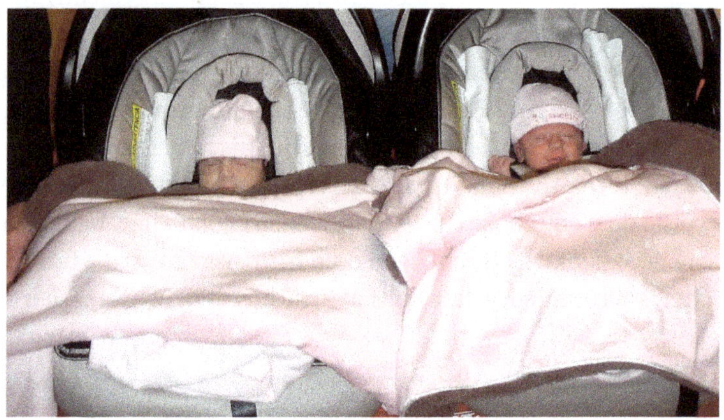

IMG 5.3

The sweetest little 35-week twin girls named Elle and Emilia were born on October 14, 2009, just a day after my own birthday. Even though Elle was about 1 pound smaller than Emilia, she did phenomenally. Of course, that's how it works a lot of the time. As nurses, we would joke that the bigger twin "hogged" all the supplies in utero; thus, when they were born, they had no idea what to do. Meanwhile, the smaller of the twins, who had to be scrappy and deal with the other twin's "intrauterine leftovers," typically did great.

Emilia's lungs weren't fully developed, so she needed oxygen for a bit—nothing long term, just enough to help her transition from her "cushy" intrauterine life. However, they were born during the H1N1 scare, so the only visitors allowed were the parents. Families would routinely get attached to their nurses, especially during times when the nurses were the only ones they could lean on when inside the NICU. Their mom said, "Because of your calming instincts, I could handle everything." If I am being honest, there is nothing calm about the NICU, so if I was giving off that vibe, I would have had to work extra hard at it because my natural instincts are to run around like a chicken with my head cut off, especially on the days when I was in charge.

Emilia ended up coming around, and Elle grew, and after just 10 days, they went home. As we prepared them for discharge, the mom asked me to be her personal nanny. I thought she was joking. I'm fairly certain I even laughed out loud, assuming she was joking, and then walked away. But get this: She wasn't joking. She truly wanted to hire me as the girls' nanny. I remember telling her, "You can't afford me. There is no way you can pay me what I make here as a nurse." But money isn't everything.

I was finishing up the last part of my master's degree at the time and was struggling to get in all the clinical hours needed, do my homework, and work a full-time (plus mandatory call) job. I had been blessed to receive a scholarship that helped with the cost of living, and so after talking to my husband, I decided to say yes.

The first day I drove to their house, I wondered, "What am I doing? This is insane. I am a NICU nurse, not a nanny." But that day and several days moving forward, I was a nanny. It was significantly easier than working in the NICU: no charting, no IV fluids, and no admissions. I just got to care for and snuggle with these sweet baby girls. The bonus was that when they slept, I got to do my homework. It was a win-win for all involved. Additionally, their mom was an attorney, so she had connections within the legal arena, and I was looking into doing "legal nurse consulting" once I graduated.

One of the most unforgettable nanny shifts was when I decided to bring my golden retriever, Sammie Sam, with me to "work." Sammie had previously gotten car sick, but the drive wasn't that far, and I figured she would be fine. Nope. She vomited *a lot* in my car—right between the middle console and the passenger seat. As I was trying to clean it up, I ripped out one of the stitches I had in my back (from a minor skin procedure), and so now, in addition to the vomit, I had blood running down my back. Normally, I would have considered "calling in," but there was nobody to take my place. So, Sammie and I went into the house to care for the girls. That also happened to be the day one of them peed all over me. They say things come in threes, which was pretty accurate that day.

After I graduated with my MSN, I got a job as an instructor at a local BSN University and needed to step down from my nanny role. The cool thing is that I found one of my students who was interested, and she took over. From there, each subsequent nanny these girls had was from a referral that initially started with me. You see, sometimes God puts opportunities on your path that make zero sense. I have found in my life that taking these opportunities have been some of the best decisions I have ever made. Their mom and I became friends, and to this day, we still talk. In fact, she helped me with some of the details of this story.

As I reflect on this story, I would be remiss not to include this next part. One day, completely out of the blue, my stepson Philip said, "Soooo ... you got your master's degree so that you could be a babysitter?" He said it very slowly, as if he was trying to put the pieces together but they just didn't make sense. Like, he could be a babysitter, and he was in junior high school. So, I just said, "Yup," and we went about our day just like any other day. To this day, when I am writing my resume, I leave off my stint as a nanny, but will always remember it in my heart.

Reflection Questions

1. How would you have responded to the mother asking you to be her nanny?
2. In your opinion, were there ethical reasons why Valerie shouldn't have accepted this position as a nanny?

Never Let the Dads Watch

One day I was helping the pediatrician with a baby boy's circumcisions. The typical process is that the pediatrician would go to the parent rooms to get consent, and while they were doing this, the nurse would gather the supplies to complete the circumcision. Something a bit different happened this day, though. As the pediatrician came back to the nursery, he had one of the dads with him. I assumed this dad was the dad of one of the baby girls in the nursery and was just coming to pick her up, but no.

As the pediatrician came into the part of the nursery where we completed the circumcisions, he politely asked the dad to "stand over there" while we got his son ready. The dad was within listening distance, so I couldn't ask the pediatrician what I wanted to, which was "What are you thinking? This is a *terrible* idea!" So, I did my best with my eyes, and the pediatrician looked at me and said, "What? It's fine! I've had dads watch before, and they do fine."

I am not sure if you have personally witnessed a circumcision being performed, but it is intense. There is a clamp placed tightly around the head of the baby boy's penis. Then the foreskin is removed with a scalpel—a scalpel. There is bleeding. There is crying. It's not really something I want to see, and these kids aren't mine. I wondered how the dad would do, and he did exactly how I thought. The moment the pediatrician clamped down the instrument on his son's penis and got out the scalpel, the dad passed out—cold, right on the floor. Except, I am the one holding the baby for the procedure, so I can't help him, and there is nobody else in the nursery. Super.

I still remember the pediatrician saying, "Just leave him there. You can get him to come around after we're done." I was furious. I remember telling the pediatrician, "This is ALL. YOUR. FAULT. We *never* should have let a dad back here for this." The second the procedure was done, I got my trusty smelling salts (typically reserved for moms who pass out) and waved them under his nose. We got a wheelchair and wheeled him and the baby back to the room. Later, I remember going into the parents' room and the dad saying, "Remember me? I was the one who passed out." To which I replied, "Yes, sir. I remember, and I am pretty sure I'll never forget."

Reflection Questions

1. Should the dad have been allowed to watch the circumcision? If not, what would you have told him was the reason he shouldn't be there?
2. As the nurse in this situation, are you responsible for what happened to the father, or is the pediatrician?

Hungry for Residual?

When feeding babies with nasogastric tubes (NG), you must check the residual before feeding. This means that you attach a syringe to the NG tube and pull out any residual feeding from the baby's stomach. You do this for a few reasons. First, you want to see how well the baby is digesting their food, as high residuals signify that something isn't right with their digestion and could be a sign of a serious gastrointestinal condition. Secondly, you look at the consistency of the residual, which then helps decide if you should put it back or toss it.

I was taking care of a baby we had been keeping a close eye on related to their residual. Luckily, this was during the day, so I could just go talk to the neonatal nurse practitioner (NNP), show them the residual, and then ask them what to do. This specific incident is permanently imprinted into my mind because when I went into her office and showed her the syringe and asked her what to do, she said, with a very straight and serious face, "If you bring me residual like that again, I am going to make you eat it."

I gagged a little bit and had no idea what to say. I was just doing my job, and under no circumstances would I eat any residual, not even my own. I remember walking out like a puppy with its tail between its legs, wondering exactly how I would chart that incident. After that, I learned not to take the residual to that specific nurse practitioner. She just wanted to be told about it but didn't want to see it, which I totally understand. Looking back, I would have loved to see my face when she told me to eat it. Um, no thanks.

Reflection Questions

1. How might you have responded when confronted by the nurse practitioner, like Valerie was?
2. As a nurse, what would you do if you were told not to do something that was actually protocol to do?

From Baby to Teacher—All in the Same Room

After I graduated with my master's degree, I worked as the perinatal educator at our hospital. We were a Level III NICU, so we often transported babies from surrounding hospitals to our NICU. Part of the transport process is teaching the referring hospital how to stabilize the baby until we arrive.

I was teaching neonatal resuscitation at one of our local hospitals, and this just happened to be the hospital I was born in. I also worked there as a healthcare technician while in nursing school, so coming back was kind of nostalgic for me. As I began teaching, one of the nurses on staff asked me what my maiden name was, and after a series of questions, she put the pieces together that she was the delivery nurse at *my* delivery! She also noted that the delivery room I was teaching in was also the delivery room I was born in. While I clearly didn't remember being born, it was super cool to have that connection. Not many people get to visit the room they were born in, but that day, I did!

Reflection Questions

1. How would you have felt standing in the room you were born in?
2. Think back to a time when something happened like this "full-circle" story. What stands out to you about that moment?

It's Hotter Than You Think

When I started as a nurse in 1999, we had just gotten a brand-new shipment of infant warmers, and they were super snazzy. I think back to when we were so excited to get them, and they don't even begin to compare to the warmers we have in 2022. Anyway, we were really full in the NICU and had used all of our shiny new warmers when a sweet little baby girl needed one, and we didn't have it.

I called the maintenance department and asked them to please get one of our old warmers from storage and bring it to us. This specific baby had a condition that affected her hypothalamus. This was a problem because one of the roles of the hypothalamus is temperature regulation. One moment, this baby's temperature would be 102°, and then the next moment, 95°. The day I was taking care of her, it was 95°. Hence, the need for a warmer.

Once the warmer was delivered, I plugged it in and turned it on high. I also grabbed one of her sweet pink sleepers and held it up to the warmer—apparently, too close. The heat caused the outfit to melt. (These old warmers also didn't have a cage around the warming coils for safety purposes.) It was like it sucked it toward the coil and then began melting it. I involuntarily screamed and moved the baby out of the way with my other arm so that the melting outfit didn't fall onto her. However, it did melt onto my hand and arm, which burned me pretty badly. As I peeled off the melted outfit from my hand and arm, it took off layers of my skin as it bled and quickly began swelling. I ended up going to the emergency department, where they cleaned out the melted outfit and dressed the burns. I actually was off work for a few weeks until they healed because I wouldn't have been able to properly wash my hands, a necessary part of being a nurse.

Come to find out, this outfit was an outfit from the 1970s. It was a family heirloom. Super. It also was not manufactured to be flame resistant, thus the reason it instantly melted on my hand and arm. I'd like to say this was my first and only encounter with being too close to a warmer, but that's not true. Because I am short, I needed a stool when caring for babies in a warmer. One night, I was leaning over the warmer during an admission and began to smell something burning. Hum. That's odd. What would be burning in here? My hair, that's what was burning. I was too close to the warmer with my head, and it burned my hair. Tiny pieces of burnt hair fell from my head, and I gasped and probably said a few words that would not be appropriate to write in this book.

Moral of the story: The warmers are hotter than you think.

Reflection Questions

1. What stood out to you when reading this story?
2. What could Valerie have done differently to avoid getting burnt?

Medication Error Lesson

In the NICU, we would routinely run total parenteral nutrition (TPN) and lipids in the baby's IV as a way to provide them with nutrition. Sometimes it was in combination with their regular feedings, and for some babies who couldn't be fed either orally or by a feeding tube, this was their sole form of nutrition. When we would hang the TPN and lipids, we would hang them in two separate IV lines, and they would each run on their own IV pump. Typically, the rate for TPN was substantially higher than the lipid rate. In fact, a typical rate might be running TPN at 5.6 ml/hr and lipids at 0.6ml/hr. The TPN rate is almost ten times the rate of lipids, thus the "situation" if the rates are switched.

As a NICU nurse, we might be assigned to three babies, and all three babies would have TPN and lipids to hang, which we typically hung in the afternoon but definitely before night shift at 7:00 p.m. Not that I am making excuses, but this was something we did a lot of, and on this day, I clearly went into autopilot. I hung the TPN and lipids, put them into the pumps, set the rates, had another nurse check the rates, pushed start, and off I went. I don't know what I did after that, but it had been less than an hour before I came back to chart my hourly documentation. At that time, I realized I had switched the rates, so the lipids were running at the TPN rate and the TPN was running at the lipids rate. It's not a big deal to run TPN at the lipids rate, especially if it is just a short time, but to run the lipids at the TPN rate—well, that is a huge deal, as outlined previously in the story.

Luckily, I caught it within the first hour. This is a classic example of how you see what you expect to see. I had done these hundreds of times. So had the other nurse. We both missed it. However, it was ultimately my fault, as I was the nurse directly responsible for the baby.

As a nurse, I had a decision to make when I found the error. I could switch the rates to what they were supposed to be and do nothing, or I could report it, which ultimately meant reporting myself. I immediately stopped both infusions and notified the nurse practitioner. I also had to submit a hospital incident report disclosing the medication error.

I beat myself up over it for days, wondering how I could have allowed the error to happen. I cried on the way home, and I literally could not stop thinking about it. I was so angry at myself. However, at the end of the day, I am human, and humans make mistakes. In the field of healthcare, there are procedures we put into place to decrease the chances of error, but this was a "Swiss cheese" moment, where all the holes of the cheese, unfortunately, lined up, and the error occurred.

After this incident, I was meticulously detailed when hanging my IV fluids. I didn't just double-check them; I triple-checked them. I am thankful my error did not have lasting consequences for the baby. In fact, it was a super simple fix, and the baby's care wasn't altered in the least. In hindsight, I shouldn't have been so hard on myself. Even the best of nurses can, and will, make mistakes.

Reflection Questions

1. What would you have done if you were in Valerie's shoes when you noticed the IV rates were switched?
2. Reflect back to a "Swiss cheese" moment of your own. What could have been done differently to avoid the outcome?

Watch Out for the Tire

It was a cold, rainy, and dark morning—the kind of morning you wish you could just stay in bed. However, the calendar said I was scheduled to be the charge nurse, so sleeping in wasn't really an option. The hospital was about 20 minutes from my house, and it took about 10 minutes to park. Since I was in charge, I needed to be there 30 minutes early. I left my house at 6:00 a.m. and headed off to work at the NICU.

As I was driving on the interstate, I saw a car in front of me swerve, and in a fraction of a second, a semitruck tire appeared in the road, rim and all, directly in front of my Hyundai Santa Fe. In what was probably only a millisecond, I remembered my dad telling me never to swerve, so I hit it head-on. It was as if the accident was occurring in fast-forward and at the slowest speed, all at the same time. I remembered thinking, "This is how I am going to die."

I watched the tire hit the front of my car and then fly up and over my car. It was a miracle, really, that it didn't come straight through the windshield and hit me. To this day, I believe an angel was there and graciously guided that tire out of harm's way to the ditch. After I hit it, I lost power steering, and the car was smoking like crazy. I was assuming it was on fire. I grabbed my cell phone and called the NICU. Not 911. Not my husband. The NICU.

I talked to the charge nurse and told her what happened. I told her I was pulled onto the shoulder, but I thought the car was on fire, and I was still in it. She had another nurse call 911 from the NICU. It was basically a three-way call until they had me hang up and call 911 directly. Meanwhile, the charge nurse yelled at me to get out of the car and get far away, warning me it might "blow up." Luckily, an off-duty firefighter passed the scene and stopped. He called off the fire department, noting it was "just" the radiator that had been demolished.

I was only a few miles from home, so my husband quickly arrived to get me. The irony is that I didn't have him take me home. I had him take me to the NICU. I was the charge nurse, and I had to cover my shift. It is funny to look back and realize how I thought I could actually work that day. My car was completely totaled. It must have been the adrenaline because once I got to the NICU, I was in terrible pain. I was really dizzy and couldn't move my head from side to side. I had a concussion and severe whiplash and obviously did not work that day or several days after that either.

In hindsight, I should have called 911, but thinking back on this situation makes me smile. As a nurse, my sense of responsibility to be at work was strong. The babies and their families were counting on me, and I wasn't going to let a semitruck tire ruin my ability to be there for them—until it did.

Reflection Questions

1. Why do you think Valerie called the NICU before calling 911?
2. Have you ever gone to work with an injury or while sick? Why did you feel the need to do so?

The Dreaded Phone Call

I was working nights, and at the time, we had a neonatal nurse practitioner (NNP) scheduled 24 hours a day. The neonatologist was home on call, and you prayed you never had to call them. However, a provider had to be "in-house" at all times. So, when we got the phone call for a transport, our NNP had to go, which only meant one thing: We had to call the on-call neonatologist in from home.

We played a simple rock, paper, and scissors to decide who had to make the call, and I unfortunately lost. After saying a few choice words in my head, I made the call. He was not happy, and honestly, I wasn't either. I didn't want him to come in any more than he wanted to come in, but a hospital policy must be followed.

I was caring for a baby who was becoming more unstable by the minute, so the NNP ordered several tests before she left. Those tests came back, which meant the neonatologist would have to look at them. There was, unfortunately, no rock, paper, and scissors to even win. This was my responsibility. Ugh.

I remembered calling and telling him about the test results, and there was just silence on the other end of the phone. Perfect. Did he fall back asleep? Was he ignoring me? What is happening? So, I said something like, "Are you there?" to which he yelled, "Of course, I'm here!" and then hung up on me. This was turning out to be a really special night.

Within minutes, he was in the NICU, stomping toward the baby's bedside with the results in hand. He came toward me, smacking the report documents into his other hand, screaming, "Who ordered these tests??!!" I just stood there. I had no idea what to do. He kept coming toward me to the point where I had to start backing up because he was so close—until I couldn't back up anymore because of the baby's ventilator. I mustered up my very best "baby backbend" to try to get farther away from him because as he was yelling, spit was coming out of his mouth and onto me.

The moment the first piece of spit hit my face, I lost it. I immediately stood straight up and then began walking toward him to where he now had to back up. I sternly but respectfully told him, "Clearly, I did not order the labs. I can't order labs. I just did what the NNP ordered. If you have a problem with it, talk to her. But our job right now is to take care of this baby." He looked at me, nodded his head, and said, "Okay." Wait, what? Just okay? No more yelling? I waited, and the yelling never came. Together, we cared for the baby, who ultimately got better. After that night, I was just a little less scared when dealing with him, and nobody ever spit on my face again.

Reflection Questions

1. What first comes to mind after reading this story?
2. Have you been in a situation where you had to advocate for yourself? If so, how did you manage it?

The Unimaginable Cry

Babies who are born to moms who have been using drugs have a very distinct and yet unimaginable cry. It really is hard to explain, but when you hear it, you know. The cry was high-pitched and shrill. These babies also tended to be inconsolable. For anyone reading this who has dealt with an inconsolable baby, you have a fraction of an idea of what it was like caring for these babies.

These babies had what is called neonatal abstinence syndrome (NAS). NAS is a group of conditions caused when a baby withdraws from certain drugs they're exposed to in the womb before birth, oftentimes opioids. There were medications we could give the babies going through withdrawal, but they didn't work that great. It always broke my heart to know how much the baby was suffering due to decisions their mom had made. With that said, the mom was also suffering, as addiction is a disease.

This was one of the hardest parts of working in the NICU, second to being with a family as their precious baby died. It was hard to watch these babies suffer from decisions they didn't get a chance to make themselves. It was hard when the parents didn't want their babies, and it was hard when they did want them, as we feared for the safety of the baby. There were babies we had to send home in less-than-optimal situations, which weighed heavily on our hearts. I would often think about these families and pray that they would be able to find the best path for them and their babies.

As NICU nurses and nurses in general, we treat each patient with dignity and respect, even those whose decisions we disagree with, and this was the case with these babies. The interesting part was that the moms almost expected us to judge them. But what they received from us was nothing short of compassion—compassion for them and compassion for their baby. At the end of the day, life is hard, and we all cope differently. I cannot imagine what it would be like to walk a day in their shoes. I am thankful for the upbringing I was blessed to receive and pray for those less fortunate.

Reflection Questions

1. What is the first thing that comes to mind after reading this story?
2. Reflect on your feelings toward the mothers of babies with NAS. How might you respond if caring for a baby with NAS, specifically related to their parents?

Don't Text and Drive

We had a teen mom who delivered the sweetest little 24-week baby girl named Macey (name changed for privacy). Macey was a fighter. She had coded many times throughout her stay in our NICU—too many times to count. One day, when she was about 6 months old, she coded, and this time we couldn't bring her back. I cannot begin to express how hard it is, as a nurse, to see a baby die after a long resuscitation. It is our job to save them, and a part of me always felt like a failure, even though I logically knew it was nothing I had done wrong.

I took care of Macey a lot and really became close with her parents. After she died, they specifically asked for one of Macey's other primary nurses and me to attend the visitation and funeral. They knew we had spent a lot of time with her and wanted us to speak at the visitation. We both scheduled the day off and went. I didn't want to go. I knew it would be hard. But who really ever wants to go to a visitation, especially that of a baby? But we went because it was the right thing to do.

I struggled to find the funeral home, and this was back in the day when to send a text, you had to multitap, which means you had to physically press the numbers until the letter popped up that you needed. (Side note: Thank God for technology.) I was driving on the right side of a one-way street. I was also distraught, as I still had not figured out what I would say, and we were close to being late because we were lost. From the corner of my eye, I saw the sign for the funeral home. I quickly grabbed my phone and texted the nurse I knew was a few cars behind me and then turned left toward the funeral home. It is as if it all happened simultaneously: the text, the turn, the crash. Remember, I was on a one-way street in the right lane, so looking to see if there was oncoming traffic did nothing about the car that was behind me in the left lane.

Luckily, none of us were injured, but my car was pretty beaten up, as was theirs. We both pulled over to assess the damage. Even though I was tearful, they were still screaming at me about how I should have been paying attention. This screaming fit seemed to go on for longer than I was expecting, and had I not been so distraught, I probably would have *actually* been listening. Still, all I could think about was that there was no way I would let these parents down and be late to sweet Macey's visitation.

I handed the lady my entire purse, left the keys in my car (I think it was actually still running), and told her, "Do whatever you need to do. I can't be late for Macey's visitation." And then I just walked away. I walked across the street, into the funeral home, and greeted Macey's family as if nothing had happened. It was just a car. This was more important. To this day, I have no idea what I said at that visitation, but I said something, and the family was grateful we were there.

After I basically did a "mic drop" and walked off, the other nurse briefly talked to the lady, explaining we had a visitation of a baby we had cared for and we were going to be late. Luckily, the lady had empathy for me, put my purse back in my car, shut it off, and left a kind note asking me to call her when I was done so we could exchange insurance information, which I did. I am not sure the texting led to the accident, but it certainly didn't help the situation. So, in closing, I hope a little smile comes across your face thinking back to this incident and how you, technically, shouldn't text and drive. Also, be kind to others when driving; you never know, they might be on their way to a baby's visitation and/or funeral.

Reflection Questions

1. How would you have felt when the parents in this situation asked you to speak at their daughter's funeral?
2. Have you ever encountered "road rage" against another driver? If so, would your feelings have changed if you knew they were on their way to a baby's visitation and funeral?

#MeToo

I worked as a waitress at a small "mom-and-pop" restaurant in my hometown in high school and college. Being a waitress is a job I feel everyone should have to do at some point in their life. The lessons I learned from that job far extended the ten-cent tips I was occasionally given. One of the key lessons I learned at that job was how to navigate men being sexually inappropriate with me.

We had a long table in the middle of the restaurant where the beloved "coffee drinkers" would sit. They were there every morning at 6:00 a.m., waiting for us to open the door. I remember thinking I would give anything to be back in bed, and these guys are consciously choosing to get up and be here. I suppose, in hindsight, they were coming for the comradery and, for some of them, to grab the waitress's butt occasionally.

Over the years, I fielded many inappropriate comments from these older men. Some were so kind and would stand up for me, telling the others to "knock it off," but unfortunately, it never really helped. I grew to realize it was just part of the job, which, in hindsight, is really sad.

When I graduated from nursing school, I was overjoyed for many reasons, but a huge one was that I wouldn't have to work as a waitress any longer—specifically, I would no longer have to endure the coffee table situations. Little did I know that I would be walking into a similar yet worse situation.

The first encounter occurred when I was on orientation in the postpartum unit. The MD had asked me to "walk with him" to the patient's room, which I thought was odd because no other MD had asked me to do that. But I did it because he was the MD, and in my mind, as a nurse, I was supposed to do whatever he said.

He put his hand on my butt as we walked down the hall. I literally could not believe what was happening. I tried moving over, and he just moved with me, continuing to keep his hand on my butt. He removed it just as we walked into the patient's room. Once in the room, I found a way to "escape" and go back to the nurses station, luckily by myself. Once I got there, I told one of the nurses who had been working there for years what had happened. Her reply shocked me. She said, "Yup, you are his type. Get used to it." I was like, "Excuse me?!?! There is no way I am getting 'used to' that." She told me it was typical for this MD and that nothing would change even if I reported it. She recommended I "just suck it up." I consulted another nurse, and she gave me the same response, except she added, "It should make you feel good. He only does it to the pretty nurses."

I had only been working there for a few weeks. I didn't know what to do, so I did nothing. I tried dodging him every time he came onto the unit, and luckily, he never went to the nursery, so that was my haven. In hindsight, I definitely should have reported it. Even as I write this, I am upset with myself for not reporting him, but I am also trying to provide myself grace. This occurred in 1999, years before the #MeToo movement was ever heard of. I had promised myself, though, if it happened again with a different MD, I would report it.

Well, interestingly enough, I had that opportunity. We had medical residents who worked in postpartum and the newborn nursery. As a part of their residency, they were required to be in our unit for six months. One of the residents and I got along really well. He was a super cool guy—until he wasn't. He knew I was married; in fact, we had talked about my wedding and upcoming honeymoon many times. He had made occasional "flirty" comments to me, but I just blew them off. I played it off as "boys will be boys" and was thankful he wasn't grabbing my butt. He overheard me talking about how I get motion sickness and how I wasn't sure what I would do on the honeymoon cruise not to get sick. He pulled me aside and told me he had an idea for how to help. He said, "Why don't you come to my office for a 'private' appointment? You give me what I need, and then I will give you whatever you need." I replied, "What are you talking about?" He said, "You know," as he smiled and winked. Eww. I remember replying, "I am not doing that, and you will not talk to me like that again." One of the other nurses overheard our conversation. She recommended I report him, but I told her I had it under control that and if he did it again, I would.

Fast forward a few months when I was in the newborn nursery, just several screaming babies and me. He walked in and said he needed me to get one of the babies under the warmer so he could assess them. I found it quite odd because babies in the nursery can hold their temperature just fine. They don't need to be in the warmer. But I did it because that is what he wanted.

Once in the warmer, the resident asked for my infant stethoscope. I told him it was mine; we had several others he could use. He reached across the warmer, grabbing mine off my chest while simultaneously grabbing my breast, and said, "I want this one," and did that same disgusting wink. I took a deep breath and told him what he did was inappropriate, and he just smiled, shrugged his shoulders, and then went on to do the baby's assessment.

I knew in my mind that I was going to report him. I just wasn't sure how. I also couldn't leave the newborn nursery right then, as I was the only nurse staffing the unit. It was also around midnight, so there was likely nobody in human resources (HR) to talk to. This was also before we really used email, so I sat in the nursery that night and festered about it. On a break, I talked to one of the other nurses, asking them how I should report it. I had a plan, but that plan changed once I received a call from the attending MD supervising the residents. He said he needed to talk to me ASAP. I had no idea how he knew because I hadn't reported anything.

In retrospect, one of the nurses overheard me talking about it to the other nurse, and she took it upon herself to call the attending right then and there. And honestly, I am thankful she did. I had committed to reporting him but wasn't really sure what the next steps would be. After talking with me, he told me he would speak to the resident and require him to write me a formal letter of apology and apologize face to face. If he didn't do those two things, he would be asked to leave the residency program.

I vividly remember telling him, "No way. I do not want to talk to him about it. He can write me a letter, but I don't want to see him again, much less talk to him about it." The attending then told me that the "wheels were already in motion" and to expect to hear from him soon. I found this to be very interesting. I was the "victim" in the situation, yet I did not even have a say in how it would be resolved.

I saw the resident walking down the hallway toward me, and I cringed. He said, "I need to talk with you privately." I quickly replied, "I am not going anywhere private with you. We can talk in the nurses lounge." So, he followed me into the nurses lounge, and we sat at the table. Before he could say a word, he began to cry, which really took me off guard. I just sat there, speechless.

He finally started talking and begged me to let his attending know he had spoken to me and that this was all resolved because he couldn't get "kicked out" of the program. He slid a piece of paper across the table and noted that now I could let the attending know. He had met all of the "requirements." The irony was that he wasn't even sorry. Or at least it didn't appear so. He was just worried about losing his place in the residency program. I wanted it all to be over, so I told him I would call the attending and let him know he had done what was required. As soon as he left the nurses lounge, I called the attending and let him know. The attending then let me know that he was transferring the resident off our floor so I wouldn't have to interact with him anymore.

This resident ultimately graduated from his residency and began working at our hospital—luckily, not in my department. I would see him from time to time around the hospital. Most times, we avoided eye contact and went about our day. I often wondered if he had done the same thing to other women or if it was just me. I hoped I was the first and last nurse he was inappropriate with.

Looking back, I am disappointed with how I managed these situations. I would confront them immediately if the same things happened to me today that happened back then. But you see, those situations helped to make me who I am today. I am also hopeful that women today feel more empowered to not tolerate sexual harassment. The time of "doing whatever the MD says," even if it is sexually inappropriate, is, I hope, over.

Reflection Questions

1. What are your thoughts about how Valerie handled these situations? What would you have done differently?
2. Do you think sexual harassment still occurs toward nurses today? If so, why do you think that?

The Nightmare of Moving From Paper to Electronic Charting

When I started in the NICU, we charted on paper. Absolutely nothing was electronic, which really, in 2023, is simply inconceivable. When the time came for us to move to the electronic health record (EHR), we knew it would be a lot of work. Change is never easy. In fact, before our official "go-live" date, two of our more experienced nurses retired early. They said they hated computers and just couldn't handle the change. If I was in their shoes, I probably would have retired too.

To add to the fun, we had 16 hours of mandatory training for this new EHR. As we prepared for our go-live date, we increased staffing because on the first few days of implementation, we had the "opportunity" to chart on paper and on the computer, which would take significantly more time. I was the lucky one to be in charge on the first 2 go-live days. Let me tell you, I have worked some horrible days in the NICU, but none of them compared to these 2 days of going live with our EHR.

For anyone reading this, I am sure you are wondering, "What's the big deal?" But it was a big deal. The first round of EHR was not made specifically for our NICU. It was hard to figure out where to chart stuff, and none of it matched our current way of charting. Several nurses throughout the day began refusing to chart on the computer and instead went back to paper charting. It was mass chaos, and in the middle of it all were critically ill babies we were caring for.

I finally went to the person in charge of the EHR, letting him know that the way the charting was within the EHR wasn't going to work. I explained how we cared for the babies and needed to document things accordingly. To this day, I can clearly remember his response, which was, "Then change the way you care for the babies to adapt to the charting." I had previously been trying to "toot" the EHR horn, but not anymore. My response was probably harsher than it should have been but went something like, "Let me tell you what, *sir*. We will not change how we care for our babies to match your charting. Your charting will change to match how we care for our babies. Period." A nurse's job is to advocate for their patients, and advocate I did!

I saw a few nurses in the background give me air high-fives. We were drowning, and it was my job to try and save us. I ended up talking to the head person for the hospital-wide go-live, and he agreed to alter the software to be more like our current form of charting, which also matched how we actually cared for the babies. We were able to put one of our NICU nurses on the EHR team to provide feedback, and the second version was substantially better than the first. Thank God.

The other interesting thing was that now providers would have to put in their own orders, and we would actually be able to read them. Before, they were handwritten and a struggle to read. Also, before if we called in the middle of the night, they would give us verbal orders, which we would then have to write. Not anymore. It would be 100% their responsibility to put them in. So, the first time a provider gave me an order and asked me to put it in, I pushed back. I said, "Nope, I can't. I am not allowed anymore to put in a physician order." All the hell of going through the go-live was suddenly all worth it at that exact moment.

Who would have thought that changing from paper to electronic charting would be such a nightmare? But nightmare it was!

Reflection Questions

1. Why do you think it was such a nightmare to move from paper to electronic charting?
2. What do you see as the pros and cons of electronic charting?

Sir, May I Please Have Some Space?

At the hospital I worked at, the NICU nurses would sometimes get called to other units to start IVs that nobody else could get. The problem is that we were usually called after several other nurses had tried and were unsuccessful. This is never a good scene to walk into, and also carries much responsibility for us to "get it" on the first stick.

I was the charge nurse the day we got the request from the emergency department (ED) to start an IV on a "difficult baby," which meant I was the one who had the "opportunity" to go. As I arrived in the ED, I could hear the dad yelling from the room about how "this NICU nurse better get it on the first attempt." I stopped in my tracks and considered going back to the NICU and either ignoring the request or having someone else go in my place. Unfortunately, the ED nurse had already seen me and waved me toward the room. Busted.

I walked in and introduced myself to the family. The dad, who was also a surgeon at our hospital, got in my face and told me they had already tried 13 times and if I couldn't guarantee to get it the first time, to go get another nurse. I honestly thought for about a millisecond of this gift he had offered me to go and get another nurse. That would have been the easier thing—for me, at least. However, I was the charge nurse, and ultimately, this was my responsibility.

As I gathered the supplies to start the IV, the dad was standing really close. When I began looking for sites on his baby's arm, he was so close that he was actually touching me. This is when I realized that it was no wonder other nurses couldn't get it if this was what they had to endure. So, I very plainly and calmly stepped back and said, "Sir, may I please have some space? I am one of the best IV starters in the NICU, but my chances of getting this IV are cut in half with you hovering over me." I was trying to let him know that I was competent at my job but that his presence was making me less competent by the second. Also, in full disclosure, while I was good at starting IVs, there were plenty of other nurses who were good as well. I was simply trying to set the stage for him that one of the "best" was here, and he needed to back off and let her do her job. In saying this, I also reaffirmed to myself that "I got this."

The look he gave me was priceless. I am confident most people don't push back with him, especially regarding his newborn infant. He looked me in the eyes, nodded his head slightly, mumbled under his breath, "You better get it," and then walked out of the room. No pressure. Nope, none at all. So, I found the best little vein I could, and with another nurse helping to hold the arm, I got it. I have never been so happy to see blood return in my life! But seeing blood return is just the first step. You have to get the tape perfect, and it has to actually flush once everything is in place. And flush it did.

The nurse hollered out to the hallway, "She got it!" while I allowed a sigh of relief to flow throughout my body. I thought, "Okay, I can breathe again. Exhale, Valerie." The dad came in, didn't say a word, but gave me a nod of approval when he saw the IV in place. I walked out, charted the IV, and with a smile on my face from ear to ear, went back to the NICU. After this day, when I would see the surgeon in the hallway, he would give me that same nod—no words, just the nod. And sometimes, a nod is better than a thousand words, especially this time.

Reflection Questions

1. How might you have handled the situation when the surgeon got in your face?
2. How might stressful situations impact a nurse's ability to do their job?

The Kitten Catastrophe

I was driving on the interstate on my way to work when I noticed cars swerving in front of me. I could tell they were swerving to miss something on the road but couldn't tell what it was. Once I got closer, I realized what they were swerving from: kittens. There was an entire litter of kittens trying to cross the interstate. I tried swerving too (which, according to my dad, I should never do) but felt my car hit one of the kittens. I screamed in horror at the catastrophe occurring in front of my eyes and immediately began pulling over to the shoulder. I suppose, to some people, it wouldn't be a big deal, but I love animals, especially puppies and kittens!

I quickly got out of my car to see if I could help the kitten. There were probably eight of them scattered around the interstate, and two of them were right on the side of the shoulder. The ones on the road had already died, but the ones on the shoulder were barely alive. I immediately went to action, trying to figure out how to save them.

As I leaned down to pick one of them up, a semitruck passed by me. If I would have reached my hand out, I could have touched the wheels. I was *way* too close to the interstate. I was clearly not thinking straight. I stepped back, took a deep breath, and reminded myself to be careful. My life was more valuable than a kitten's life.

I noticed blood coming from the one kitten's mouth, nose, and ears. Before I could pick him up, he died. The other kitten was making a screeching sound. To this day, I can still hear it. I picked him up and held him close to me, and as if he could understand me, I told him I would do everything I could to save him. It was as if I was at work, except I was on the side of the interstate, and these were kittens, not babies.

I had initially left home early so I would be early for work, but now I was going to be late for work. I called the NICU to let them know what was going on. I was crying so hard I could barely talk. They assumed something tragic had happened to my family and were relieved to hear it was "just" kittens, but I still was really upset. I called the emergency vet clinic and let them know I was on my way, but before I could start driving again, the last kitten died in my arms.

I sat in my car and sobbed. I had no idea what to do with the kitten. I couldn't take it to work with me, and it didn't feel right just tossing it out on the road. I would like to say I buried it and then made a little cross out of sticks, placing it over the ground where I buried him. But I honestly don't remember. I know I didn't take him to work, and I know I didn't just leave him on the side of the road, but my memory is just blank as to what I did next, other than remembering going to work.

When I arrived at work, I remember being about an hour late. This meant that the night shift nurse had to stay over until I got there. Luckily, she loved cats and had an extra dose of grace for me. I was a hot mess, to say the least. My makeup was smeared everywhere. My hair was a mess. And I couldn't stop crying. I just kept seeing the kittens all over the interstate, feeling my car hit one of them, and hearing the screeching of the suffering kitten. As a nurse, you are supposed to leave behind whatever happens at home. If I was grading myself on how well I did with that task on that specific day, I'd give myself a big fat F.

Reflection Questions

1. What first comes to your mind after reading this story?
2. If in a similar situation, would you have pulled over? If so, what would you have done?
3. If you had been the night nurse who had to stay on, would you have had a similar level of empathy?

How Much Epi?

It was the middle of the night, and one of the babies was coding. Our neonatal nurse practitioner (NNP) was in-house and immediately came to the bedside to direct the code. Other units have teams that come in and manage the code, but in the NICU, we ran our own. The baby who was coding was not my patient, but a code is an "all hands-on deck" situation.

My role in this specific code was to draw up medications. Seems easy enough, right? Except the code team needed the drugs, like, "yesterday," and it takes a bit of time to draw them up, label them, and hand them over. Medication errors are never a good thing, especially during a code. The NNP then asked us to call the neonatologist, who was at home. Somehow, I got that job too.

I looked through the Rolodex (yes, the Rolodex), found his number, and called. After waking him up, I briefed him on the situation. I was then the middleman between the NNP and the neonatologist—a spot I would prefer never to be in.

The neonatologist began giving orders, which I tried to quickly write down, then draw up, then hand to the code team. Words cannot describe the amount of pressure I was under. I loved working in the NICU but hated this part of the job. The neonatologist was giving me orders, one of which I couldn't understand, so I asked him again. I still didn't understand, and so I reluctantly asked a third time. He yelled the answer back to me, as if talking louder would actually help.

See, this was the thing: I wasn't having a hard time understanding the content of what he said; I was having a hard time understanding how to do what he wanted me to do. The dosage of the resuscitation medication wasn't lining up with his order. The code team was yelling at me to get them the drugs. This sucked.

So, I told the neonatologist, "Just tell me how much to draw up in the syringe." I knew I would get yelled at but did it anyway. What he said didn't make any sense, and I refused to draw up the incorrect amount. I was also a fairly new NICU nurse and so didn't have the experience to fall back on. After I asked, there was a fair amount of silence, and he said something like "0.5 ml" So, that's what I did. I drew it up, labeled it, and handed it to the code team. I then got back on the phone and waited for my "talking to" about not understanding what he was saying, but it never came. We ultimately ended up successfully resuscitating the baby, who went on to eventually go home with his family.

That next morning, when he came into the hospital, I was expecting to get yelled at—but nothing. He never said a word about it. I was floored. I wonder back if he just thought the whole thing was a dream. I don't know, and I will never know because there was no way I was ever going to bring it up to him.

Reflection Questions

1. How would you have reacted if you were in Valerie's shoes?
2. Why was it particularly important to have clear communication in this situation?

You See What You Expect to See

Back in the early 2000s, we charted on paper. We also did not have scanners, so we simply got the medication out of the Omnicell (the machine that held all the medications), checked it against the paper MAR (Medication Administration Record), and gave it. We also had a small refrigerator within the Omnicell, as some medications needed to be refrigerated. These medications were all just in little bins in the refrigerator, so you typed in the medication you needed, the fridge door popped open, you got what you needed, and then you went to give it.

That same process happened one night as the nurse went to get a "normal saline" flush from the refrigerator. The baby she was caring for had an IV but no fluids running through it, so it intermittently had to be flushed to stay patent (open). But something was odd about this vial. Usually, the flush vial held 5 ml of fluid, and this nurse could only pull up around 2.5 ml of fluid. The order was to flush 5 ml of fluid, which meant she was going to have to get another vial, which was also odd. You see, as a nurse, or anybody really, when too many things are coming up "odd," you should consider checking what is going on, and luckily, that is what the nurse did that night.

The normal saline vials looked identical to the morphine sulfate vials, just a slightly different color cap. Both were made up by pharmacy. I often thought that somebody should do something to make them look less similar, but before this night, that hadn't happened. The nurse ended up going back and looking closer at the vial to discover that she had in fact drawn up 2.5 ml of morphine sulfate, not normal saline. To give you a frame of reference as to why this would have been a likely "sentinel event" is because our usual dosage of morphine sulfate would have been around 0.25 ml or even less, meaning that 2.5 ml would have been 10 times the dose. Additionally, morphine has to be pushed through the IV at a very slow rate, and normal saline is pushed fairly quickly. The consequences could have been fatal unless we could figure it out fast enough and give Narcan (a drug that can treat a drug opioid overdose). However, she wouldn't have been expecting a narcotic overdose, so there's no way to tell what might have happened, other than to say it wouldn't have been good.

As a nurse, you think to yourself, "I won't be the nurse to make a medication error." I mean, who wants to be *that* nurse? But this nurse didn't set out to make a potential medication error. She got in the refrigerator like every other night (muscle memory) and, in a dimly lit area, pulled out what she thought was normal saline. Honestly, I bet if there were 5 ml in that vial, she never would have questioned it.

Luckily, the nurse was brave enough to admit her error. Because of that, our hospital did a "root cause analysis" where, collectively, we looked for the underlying (root cause) of the potential error. The nurse was not disciplined but applauded for her bravery in reporting the incident. After that, the normal saline was moved into prefilled syringes, and the dosage of morphine was decreased to 0.5 ml per vial—all good changes to improve patient safety.

Fast forward to electronic charting, where we scan every medication with every patient ID band. The scanning would have caught it; however, back then, there was no such thing. To think back on that time is wild. Like, how did we not make more mistakes? I have a love/hate relationship with the electronic health record, but when it comes to catching mistakes, it is truly invaluable!

Reflection Questions

1. Imagine you just caught yourself before administering a fatal dose of a medication to your patient. How would you feel?
2. Who do you think would be most responsible, the nurse who administered the medication or the people who failed to make the two medications easily distinguishable?
3. What are your key takeaways from this story?

What Was the Temperature Again?

In the summer, we would have nurse interns in the NICU. These interns were nursing students who had completed a minimum of 1 year of nursing school. They were then paired with a nurse on the unit. This was such a great learning opportunity for these soon-to-be nurses. Sometimes clinical in nursing school was only 4–6 hours, but these interns followed our shifts to see what 12-hour shifts were really like—sort of a fully immersive experience. And they got paid. Bonus!

I was assigned one of the interns whom I absolutely loved working with. She caught on so quickly and excelled in her role. But at the end of the day, regardless of how well she was catching on, she still was not a licensed registered nurse and was only able to work if she was working under the direct supervision of a licensed registered nurse. As a nurse, even if you delegate something, it is ultimately still your responsibility to ensure it is done correctly. It is *a lot* of responsibility.

I had observed her several times doing NG (nasogastric) feedings, which we often did when babies couldn't get in the required amount of feeding by solely bottle or breastfeeding. She also knew that before starting a feeding, we had to check the baby's temperature (ensuring it was at least 97.4°). I assumed she had checked the temperature, that it was high enough, and then started the NG feeding, but something in my gut was off. So, I asked her, "You checked that kid's temp, right?" to which she replied, "Yup." Still, something was off, so I asked her if she remembered what it was. She replied,

"95.3°" and I about fell out of my chair. I asked her to repeat herself, and unfortunately, she said the same thing.

I immediately went to the baby, stopped the feeding, and moved them into a warmer to get them warmed up. You see, if the body is focusing on staying warm, then it cannot focus on digestion, which could potentially lead to a serious gastrointestinal issue, like necrotizing enterocolitis. This baby ended up being totally fine, but what a great reminder to me as a nurse to be clear with my instructions. We don't just check the temperature before the feeding; we also evaluate what that temperature is to decide if feeding is okay or not. Evaluation is a key role of a registered nurse. So is delegation.

Reflection Questions

1. If a nurse delegates something to someone who is beyond competent to do the task, is the task still the nurse's responsibility? If so, why?
2. How would you have reacted with the nurse intern if you were in Valerie's shoes?

Intoxicated Coworker

I was working the night shift and getting ready to give report on a critically ill baby. The nurse I was giving the report to seemed a bit "off." As I talked to her, I noticed her breath smelled like alcohol. I also noticed a bar stamp on her hand. I had no idea what to do. I remembered learning about this in nursing school but never assumed it would happen to me. As if on autopilot, I gave report out loud while considering options in my head.

I considered this nurse my friend but also had an obligation to the patient she was going to be caring for. I stopped giving report and, as quietly as possible, asked her if she had been drinking. She said she had gone out the night before but was home in "plenty of time." Upon questioning her further, I learned she had stayed out drinking until 3:00 a.m. and was now getting report at 6:45 a.m., which was not enough time. I remember telling her that she could tell the manager, or I would, but either way, I couldn't let her care for this baby.

She was unhappy with me, to put it mildly, and reiterated that she was fine, but I knew she wasn't. She finally went and told the manager. The manager had her go into our empty rooming out room to "sleep it off" and then go home. I don't know if she was formally disciplined, and it's technically not my business. It was, however, my responsibility to protect the patient. To this day, nobody knows why she left that day. I had told the other nurses she wasn't feeling well. To my knowledge, it never happened again.

As a nurse, it is our job to advocate for our patients, and sometimes that is uncomfortable. You see, the easier thing would have been to ignore the situation, give the report, and go home. But “easy” and “nursing” rarely go hand and hand.

Reflection Questions

1. How might you have responded to the nurse in this story?
2. What repercussions do you think there should have been for the nurse who came to work intoxicated?

If You Don't Know, Ask

In the NICU and in the newborn nursery, we used to have to draw up our own IV antibiotics. For example, ampicillin came in powder form in a vial. As the nurse, we would add IV sterile water to the vial of powder, mix it up, and draw out the dosage we needed using a filter needle. Throughout my 14 years in the NICU, I did this hundreds of times.

One day, I was caring for a baby and saw the newborn nursery nurse come to the NICU to get the supplies to give ampicillin. I also saw her get into the formula cabinet and get out a bottle of oral sterile water, which was routinely used to mix formula. I thought to myself, "That's odd," but went about caring for the baby. Out of the corner of my eye, I saw the nurse put a syringe into the *oral* sterile water and then went to put that water into the vial of ampicillin—except, you can't do that. There is a difference between sterile water for oral use and sterile water for IV use.

I calmly stopped what I was doing and went to the medication preparation area to talk with her. I said something like, "So, you've got to give ampicillin in the nursery?" She gave me the strangest look and said, "Yup." So, now I need to tell her that what she did was wrong but in a way that doesn't make me seem like a "bizzo" or like I was watching her. So, I said, "Are you using this oral sterile water for formula?" She said, "No, I used it for the ampicillin." I was hoping that while we were talking about it, the error would start to click in her mind, but it didn't. So, I pulled out the container of oral sterile water and then got a vial of sterile water for IV use and showed her how the oral container says specifically, "For oral use only. Not for IV use." Then I stopped talking as the "Aha!" look came across her face. She was new to the nursery and hadn't ever had to give ampicillin and planned on just figuring it out on her own. She thanked me for telling her in a kind way and not belittling her for doing it incorrectly. I was just glad I was there to see what she was doing so that I could catch it.

The moral of the story is, if you don't know, ask. Ego has no place in the NICU—or healthcare period.

Reflection Questions

1. Have you ever been in a situation where you had to step in and correct someone's mistake? How did it make you feel?
2. Had Valerie not seen the mix-up, what do you think would have happened?
3. Do you think Valerie reacted properly? Would you have done anything differently?

Please Don't Take the Baby

I was working the night shift and caring for a baby who was basically on autopilot. He was what we called a "feeder-grower." This meant that he was stable but still too small to go home and likely hadn't really gotten the hang of how to eat yet. He was in an isolette to keep him warm but otherwise extremely stable. The NICU babies were typically on an every-3-hour feeding schedule, so between feedings, our goal was to leave them alone so they could sleep and grow. Something was different that night, though. For some reason, I went to his bed early to check on him, and I was so thankful I did.

He looked terrible. His color was greyish, and he was extremely lethargic. When I went to turn him over, he barely moved at all. Had he not been on a continuous cardiac monitor, I would have questioned if he was even alive. I immediately got the nurse practitioner, and we began running tests. The respiratory therapist came and drew an arterial blood gas. The results were terrible. We ended up having to put him on CPAP (continuous positive airway pressure) and considered even intubating him to put him on a ventilator.

When we fixed one thing, something else went wrong. This baby went from being super stable to being the most unstable baby in the NICU. Because it was the middle of the night, I held off on calling the parents because just as fast as he "went downhill," he got better. By morning, he was back in room air, pink as could be, acting as if nothing happened. It was baffling. So, I gave report to the day shift nurse, and she said she would call his parents a bit later in the morning to inform them of what happened.

I came back that night and was assigned the same baby. As I was getting report, the day shift nurse told me how angry the parents were that we hadn't called them. The dad was furious and walked out of the NICU, but the mom stayed behind and explained to the nurse why the dad was so upset. Apparently, the dad had a dream that his deceased father was planning to "take the baby" to be with him in Heaven. The dream went on through the night, with the dad of the baby begging his own father, "Please, don't take the baby." He woke up when his father finally agreed (in the dream) to leave his grandson alone on Earth. I mean, I cannot make this stuff up. My jaw dropped as the nurse told me this story. I don't believe in ghosts, but something inexplainable had happened the night before, and the strangeness of it all seemed to correlate with this dream.

When this same baby was moved to a crib, his parents brought in this stuffed giraffe, which played music when there was motion in front of it. To be honest, it kind of freaked me out. So, when I would care for this baby, I would purposefully turn off the giraffe and turn it around so it wasn't facing the baby or me. One night, I walked over to his crib, and the giraffe started playing. I yelled at my fellow nurses, telling them it wasn't funny. They knew it freaked me out, and this was not the time for jokes, but each of them swore it wasn't them. One of them came over and flipped over the giraffe, and the switch was off. How did it play the tune when it was off??!! I really wanted to put that thing in the trash but was already on thin ice with the family. To this day, neither the baby becoming rapidly unstable nor the random tune from the giraffe can be explained. So, you decide.

Reflection Questions

1. After reading this story, what do you think was really happening that night?
2. How can you explain that Valerie knew to go check on this baby early? Do you think it was coincidence, instinct, or something else?

PART VI

Case Studies

Intoxicated Coworker

After reading the story titled "Intoxicated Coworker" (page 179) and completing the reflection questions, please answer the following additional questions:

1. List 10 indicators of drug abuse in nursing.
2. List 10 indicators of alcohol abuse in nursing.
3. What does the Board of Nursing recommend in your state for these situations?
4. What do you do if you suspect your nursing colleague is intoxicated?
5. What are the most frequently abused substances by nurses?
6. How do nurses obtain controlled substances?
7. Why are nurses at risk for drug/alcohol abuse?

What Was the Temperature Again?

After reading the story titled "What Was the Temperature Again?" (page 177) and completing the reflection questions, please answer the following additional questions:

1. What, if anything, can be delegated in the nursing process?
2. Do guidelines for delegation vary from state to state? If so, how?
3. What are the five rights of delegation?
4. When an RN is delegating, how might it differ between delegating to an RN, LPN, and unlicensed assistive personnel?
5. What category would the nurse intern fall into from this story?
6. What are items that the RN cannot delegate?
7. The American Nurses Association (ANA) and the National Council of State Boards of Nursing (NCSBN) have published a joint statement on delegation. Review this joint statement online (https://www.nursingworld.org/practice-policy/nursing-excellence/official-position-statements/id/joint-statement-on-delegation-by-ANA-and-NCSBN/), and write your top three takeaways from the document.

Medication Error Lesson

After reading the story titled "Medication Error Lesson" (page 150) and completing the reflection questions, please answer the following additional questions:

1. As a nurse, what would you do if you noticed you had delivered a medication in error?
2. Can a nurse be reprimanded for self-disclosing their medication error?
3. What elements must be present to constitute malpractice (professional negligence)?

4. Could the situation in this story be considered malpractice (professional negligence)?
5. Do nurses routinely have malpractice coverage at the facility where they work?
6. What is a root cause analysis, and would it be necessary for this scenario?
7. What could happen to this patient if the lipids had continued to go at the TPN rate for more than a few hours?

You See What You Expect to See

After reading the story titled "You See What You Expect to See" (page 174) and completing the reflection questions, please answer the following additional questions:

1. What system errors occurred the night of this story?
2. How would this situation have been different if there were 5 ml of morphine in the vial?
3. What might have happened if the nurse had pushed the morphine instead of the normal saline?
4. Had the morphine been pushed, how would the nurse have recognized what was going on with the baby when their breathing began to slow and ultimately stop if they assumed they had pushed normal saline?
5. As a healthcare worker, how do you manage the potential error when it is human nature for us to see what we expect to see?
6. Hypothetically, had the nurse pushed the morphine and the baby died, would the nurse be held liable for malpractice?
7. What should have been reported in the root cause analysis report?

It Wasn't Supposed to Happen

After reading the story titled "It Wasn't Supposed to Happen" (page 59) and completing the reflection questions, please answer the following additional questions:

1. What is necrotizing enterocolitis (NEC), and how does it affect preterm infants?
2. What are the ethical implications of a Level III perinatal center closing (diverting to another hospital) due to space?
3. How might a patent ductus arteriosus (PDA) affect the outcome of a preterm infant?
4. As a nurse, how do you manage your own feelings when dealing with tragic situations?
5. What are your thoughts regarding Valerie's attachment to the Penn family?
6. How do you think it impacted the Penn family to have one baby home and doing well, with the other critically ill in the NICU?
7. To this day, Valerie believes Miles waited to die until she wasn't there. What are your thoughts?

There's No Heartbeat

After reading the story titled "There's No Heartbeat" (page 72) and completing the reflection questions, please answer the following additional questions:

1. What do you think happened to this baby in utero?
2. What would you have expected to see on the fetal monitor strip if the baby's condition was worsening?
3. What are the current NRP guidelines for how long to resuscitate a baby, and how do they differ from what happened in this story?
4. NRP guidelines give criteria for stopping resuscitation after a certain amount of time. As the healthcare team, what do you do if the parents ask you to continue?

5. What ethical principles would be applicable in this story, and how?
6. How would the resuscitation have changed (if at all) if the baby's parents weren't watching the entire thing?
7. What are your top three takeaways after reading this story and answering the questions above?

Just 5 More Minutes

After reading the story titled "Just 5 More Minutes" (page 106) and completing the reflection questions, please answer the following additional questions:

1. What is placenta accreta, and what are the different types of the condition?
2. What is the most severe form of placenta accreta?
3. Is there anything we can do in healthcare to prevent placenta accreta?
4. How is placenta accreta treated?
5. How do you handle tough questions from families, especially when you know the outcomes are not likely to be good?
6. Put yourself in the place of the anesthesiologist. How would you have responded when the mom asked for "5 more minutes?"
7. How can you apply what you learned from reading this story and answering the questions above to your own nursing practice?

PART VII

Reflective Journaling

1. After reading this book, my feelings about NICU nursing are ...

2. As emotions came up when reading the NICU stories, I found myself ...

3. My top three takeaways after reading this book are ...

4. Looking back through the stories, the three that stood out the most were ...

5. Things I know now that I didn't know before reading the book are ...

6. The benefits of having read this book include ...

7. The most difficult part of reading the NICU stories was ...

8. The personal characteristics I related to from the different authors and stories were ...

9. My takeaways regarding how to deal with challenging family situations are ...

10. My favorite story in the book was ...

11. The story in the book that made me smile was ...

12. The most challenging story to read was ...

13. I personally deal with grief and loss by ...

14. I would process my emotions when transitioning from the death of a patient to the birth of a new life, all on the same day by ...

15. Describe what you have learned about yourself after reading this book.

16. How can you apply your key takeaways from the book in your own life?

____

____

____

____

____

____

17. How has your view of being a NICU nurse changed, if any, since reading the book?

____

____

____

____

____

____

18. What questions/uncertainties do you still have about the NICU?

19. What are three things you are grateful for after reading this book?

PART VIII

Resources

There are several NICU resources available online, both for families and for healthcare professionals. The list below is not exhaustive, but it is a good start for those of you who might want to learn more about the NICU.

- March of Dimes: https://www.marchofdimes.org/nicu-initiatives
- Project Sweet Peas NICU Resources: https://www.nicuawareness.org/nicu-resources.html
- Hand to Hold: https://handtohold.org/
- Vermont Oxford Network: https://public.vtoxford.org/
- National Association of Neonatal Nurses: https://nann.org/
- World Health Organization Resources on Newborn Health: https://www.who.int/teams/maternal-newborn-child-adolescent-health-and-ageing/newborn-health/preterm-and-low-birth-weight

- Academy of Neonatal Nursing Recommended Links: https://www.academyonline.org/general/recommended_links.asp
- Association of Women's Health, Obstetric, and Neonatal Nurses: https://www.awhonn.org/nurse-resources/neonatal-and-newborn-care-resources/

Index

www.ingramcontent.com/pod-product-compliance
Ingram Content Group UK Ltd.
Pitfield, Milton Keynes, MK11 3LW, UK
UKHW021831270726
14058UKWH00001B/84

9 798823 308847